Jenny Lindberg

(414) ~~368-3045~~

321-0932 H

368-3045 W

2/19

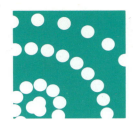

Atlas of
Regional
Anesthesia

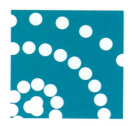

Atlas of Regional Anesthesia

David L. Brown, M.D.

Associate Professor of Anesthesiology
Mayo Medical School
Consultant
Mayo Clinic
Rochester, Minnesota

Illustrations by Jo Ann Clifford

W.B. SAUNDERS COMPANY
A Division of Harcourt Brace & Company
Philadelphia   London   Toronto   Montreal   Sydney   Tokyo

W.B. SAUNDERS COMPANY
A Division of
Harcourt Brace & Company

The Curtis Center
Independence Square West
Philadelphia, Pennsylvania 19106

Library of Congress Cataloging-in-Publication Data

Brown, David L. (David Lee)
    Atlas of regional anesthesia / David L. Brown ; illustrations by
Jo Ann Clifford.
       p.   cm.
    Includes bibliographical references and index.
    ISBN 0-7216-3177-0
    1. Conduction anesthesia—Atlases.   2. Local anesthesia—Atlases.
I. Title.
    [DNLM: 1. Anesthesia, Conduction—methods—atlases.   WO 517
B877a]
    RD84.B76   1992
    617.9'64—dc20
    DNLM/DLC   91-26484

Editor: Richard Zorab
Designer: Bill Boehm
Production Manager: Carolyn Naylor
Manuscript Editor: Wynette Kommer
Illustration Coordinator: Peg Shaw
Page Layout Artist: Terri Siegel
Indexer: Ann Cassar
Cover Designer: Michelle Maloney

ATLAS OF REGIONAL ANESTHESIA   ISBN 0-7216-3177-0

Printed in the United States of America.

Last digit is the print number: 9   8   7   6   5   4   3   2

Dedicated to

Kathryn, Sarah, and Cody

And you who think to reveal the figure of a man in words, with his limbs arranged in all their different attitudes, banish the idea from you, for the more minute your discription the more you will confuse the mind of the reader and the more you will lead him away from the knowledge of the thing described. It is necessary therefore for you to represent and describe.

LEONARDO DA VINCI
(1452–1519)

*The Notebooks of
Leonardo da Vinci,
Vol I, Ch III†*

†Translator: Edward MacCurdy
Reynal & Hitchcock, New York, 1938

Preface

Anesthesia, comprehensively administered, is a blend of art and science. The proper proportion of each is often difficult to articulate and often depends on the individuals involved. In regional anesthesia, the need to blend art with science has long been recognized and promoted. One of the principal thrusts of my effort in creating this *Atlas of Regional Anesthesia* is to utilize a heavy proportion of art (i.e., illustrations) in the "mix." I believe that these images will provide physicians with an improved understanding of the anatomy and the technical details necessary for the successful use of regional anesthesia.

Over the years my interest in regional anesthesia has led me to consult many regional anesthesia texts and atlases. Review of these books has convinced me that a large number of the illustrations have been developed from a common lineage, sometimes out of necessity but occasionally simply perpetuating the biases of this common lineage. My goal with this atlas is to combine my daily approach to the practice of regional anesthesia with an understanding of regional block anatomy. Cross-sectional anatomy is emphasized, since it is crucial to really learning regional block techniques and developing a three-dimensional concept of block anatomy. The anatomic illustrations are supplemented with newer clinical imaging views to add another perspective to these important anatomic concepts. Nevertheless, the aim throughout this work is to simplify rather than to make the images complex. For example, this text is not referenced in the classic manner, Rather, regional anesthesia references are listed in the appendix for consultation when necessary. I hope that this atlas is useful to anesthesiology trainees (residents and fellows) and to practicing anesthesiologists and other physicians interested in making regional anesthesia "work" in their practices. Throughout the *Atlas* each block has been organized around the three big P's—block *perspective*, block *placement*, and block *pearls*. The division *Perspective* is subdivided into patient selection and pharmacologic choice. The division *Placement* uses the subdivisions— anatomy, position, needle puncture, and potential problems. Finally, the division *Pearls* highlights some clinical tips to make regional anesthesia really work in clinical practice.

This *Atlas* would not have been possible without the help and encouragement of many colleagues and friends. Lewis Reines approached me years ago with the idea of a regional anesthesia atlas, and without his encouraging perspective the project probably would not have gotten off the ground. Richard Zorab deserves credit for being the major facilitator of the work. He managed to keep both the artistic and the practical issues anchored so that the project was completed. Lois Newman, Ph.D., anatomist at Thomas Jefferson University Medical School, also deserves thanks for providing a thoughtful and detailed review of the anatomy, so important to this work. Gale E. Thompson, M.D., a colleague and friend in Seattle, deserves thanks for collaborating on the concepts for the work while initial ideas were being developed. Denise J. Wedel, M.D., my colleague and friend at the Mayo Clinic, also deserves thanks for critically reviewing the text.

Perhaps most important to the book's completion was the opportunity that I had during my years in Seattle with the Virginia Mason Clinic to practice in an anesthesia department with a rich history of successfully incorporating regional anesthesia into clinical practice. Daniel C. Moore, M.D., and L. Donald Bridenbaugh, M.D., both deserve special thanks for encouraging my interest in regional anesthesia as well as for simply being friends. Another special friend who deserves thanks is Randall L. Carpenter, M.D., whose presence in the department in Seattle provided not only encouragement but also an unequaled sounding board for ideas. The organizational and secretarial skills of two coworkers and friends, Maureen Beaulieu and Barbara Hughes, were also essential to the completion of this work.

Finally and importantly, this work would not have been possible without the dedication and artistry of Jo Ann Clifford. Through her art she brings to life many concepts that I attempt to articulate but that are made so much clearer by her illustrations.

DAVID L. BROWN

Introduction

The necessary, but somewhat artificial, separation of anesthetic care into regional or general anesthetic techniques often ends with the concept that these two techniques should not or cannot be mixed. Nothing could be further from the truth. To provide comprehensive regional anesthesia care, it is absolutely essential that the anesthesiologist be skilled in all aspects of anesthesia. This concept is not original: John Lundy promoted this idea in the 1920s when he outlined his concept of "balanced anesthesia." Even before Lundy promoted this the familiar term, George Crile had written extensively on the concept of anociassociation, which was in reality the forerunner to balanced anesthesia.

It is often tempting, and quite human, to trace the evolution of a discipline back through the discipline's developmental family tree. When such an investigation is carried out for regional anesthesia, Louis Gaston Labat, M.D., often receives credit for being central in its development. Nevertheless, Labat's interest and expertise in regional anesthesia had been nurtured by Dr. Victor Pauchet of Paris, France, to whom Dr. Labat was an assistant. The real trunk of the developmental tree of regional anesthesia consists of the physicians willing to incorporate regional techniques into their early surgical practices. In Labat's original 1922 text *Regional Anesthesia: Its Technique and Clinical Application,* Dr. William Mayo in the foreword stated:

> "The young surgeon should perfect himself in the use of regional anesthesia, which increases in value with the increase in the skill with which it is administered. The well equipped surgeon must be prepared to use the proper anesthesia, or the proper combination of anesthesias, in the individual case. I do not look forward to the day when regional anesthesia will wholly displace general anesthesia; but undoubtedly it will reach and hold a very high position in surgical practice."

Perhaps if the current generation of both surgeons and anesthesiologists had kept Mayo's concept in mind, our patients would be the beneficiaries.

It appears that these early surgeons were better able to incorporate regional techniques into their practices because they did not see the regional block as the "end all." Rather, they saw it as part of a comprehensive package that had benefit for their patients. Surgeons and anesthesiologists in that era were able to avoid the flawed logic that often seems to pervade application of regional anesthesia today. These individuals did not hesitate to supplement their blocks with sedatives or light general anesthetics; they did not expect each and every block to be "100%." The concept that a block has failed unless it provides complete anesthesia without supplementation seems to have occurred when anesthesiology developed as an independent specialty. To be successful in carrying out regional anesthesia, we must be willing to get back to our roots and embrace the concepts of these early workers who did not hesitate to supplement their regional blocks. Ironically, today some consider a regional block a failure if the initial dose does not produce complete anesthesia; yet these same individuals complement our "general anesthetists" who utilize the concept of anesthetic titration as a goal. Somehow, we need to meld these two views into one that allows comprehensive, titrated care to be provided for all our patients.

As Dr. Mayo emphasized in Labat's text, it is doubtful that regional anesthesia will "ever wholly displace general anesthesia." Likewise, it is equally clear that general anesthesia will probably never be able to replace the appropriate use of regional anesthesia. One of the principal rationales for avoiding the use of regional anesthesia through the years has been that it was "expensive" in terms of operating room and physician time. As is often the case, when examined in detail some accepted truisms need rethinking. Thus, it is surprising that much of the renewed interest in regional anesthesia results from focusing on health care costs and the need to decrease the length and cost of hospitalization.

If regional anesthesia is to be incorporated successfully into a practice, there must be time for anesthesiologist and patient to discuss the upcoming operation and anesthetic prescription. Likewise, if regional anesthesia is to be effectively used, some area of an operating suite must be utilized to place the blocks prior to moving patients to the main operating room. Immediately at hand in this area, one needs both anesthetic and resuscitative equipment (regional trays, and so on), as well as a variety of local anesthetic drugs that can be used to walk along the time line of anesthetic duration. Even after successful completion of the technical aspect of regional anesthesia, an anesthesiologist's work is really just beginning. To emphasize, it is as important intraoperatively to use appropriate sedation as it was preoperatively while the block was being administered.

Contents

1

Local Anesthetics and
Regional Anesthesia Equipment

Far too often, those unfamiliar with regional anesthesia regard it as complex because of the long list of local anesthetics available and the many descriptions of varied techniques. Certainly unfamiliarity with any subject will make it look complex; thus the goal throughout this book is to simplify regional anesthesia rather than add to its complexity.

One of the first steps in simplifying regional anesthesia is to understand the two principal decisions necessary in prescribing a regional technique. First, the appropriate technique needs to be chosen for the patient, the procedure, and the physicians involved. Second, the appropriate local anesthetic must be matched to patient, procedure, regional technique, and physicians.

The following chapters will detail how to integrate these concepts into your practice.

Drugs

It is evident that not all procedures and physicians are created equal, at least regarding the amount of time needed to complete an operation. Thus, if anesthesiologists are to utilize regional techniques effectively, they must be able to choose a local anesthetic that lasts the "right amount of time." To do this, it is necessary to develop an understanding of walking across the local anesthetic time line from the shorter-acting to the longer-acting agents (Fig. 1–1).

All local anesthetics are composed of the basic structure of aromatic end, intermediate chain, and amine end (Fig. 1–2). This basic structure is subdivided clinically into two classes of drugs: (1) The amino esters possess an ester linkage between the aromatic end and intermediate chain. These drugs include cocaine, procaine, 2-chloroprocaine, and tetracaine (Figs. 1–3 and 1–4). (2) The second type of local anesthetic is the amino amides, which contain an amide link between the aromatic end and intermediate chain. These drugs include lidocaine, mepivacaine, prilocaine, ropivacaine, bupivacaine, and etidocaine (Fig. 1–4).

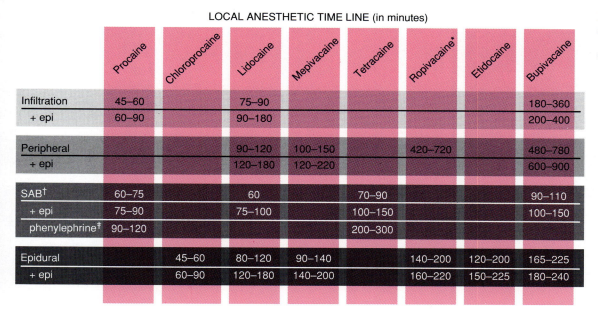

LOCAL ANESTHETIC TIME LINE (in minutes)

	Procaine	Chloroprocaine	Lidocaine	Mepivacaine	Tetracaine	Ropivacaine*	Etidocaine	Bupivacaine
Infiltration	45–60		75–90					180–360
+ epi	60–90		90–180					200–400
Peripheral			90–120	100–150		420–720		480–780
+ epi			120–180	120–220				600–900
SAB†	60–75		60		70–90			90–110
+ epi	75–90		75–100		100–150			100–150
phenylephrine‡	90–120				200–300			
Epidural		45–60	80–120	90–140		140–200	120–200	165–225
+ epi		60–90	120–180	140–200		160–220	150–225	180–240

*Not available for clinical use at time of publication

†Subarachnoid block

‡For lower extremity surgery

Figure 1–1 Local anesthetic time line (length in minutes of surgical anesthesia)

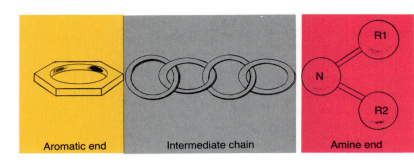

Figure 1–2 Basic local anesthetic structure

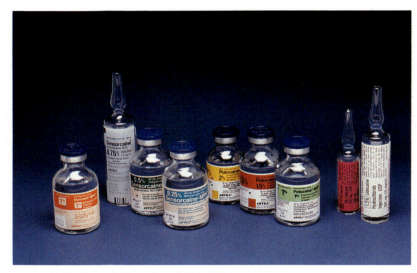

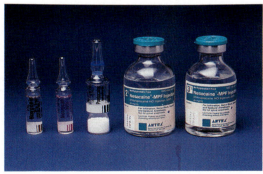

Figure 1–3 Local anesthetics commonly used in the United States

Figure 1–4 Chemical structure of commonly used amino ester and amino amide local anesthetics.

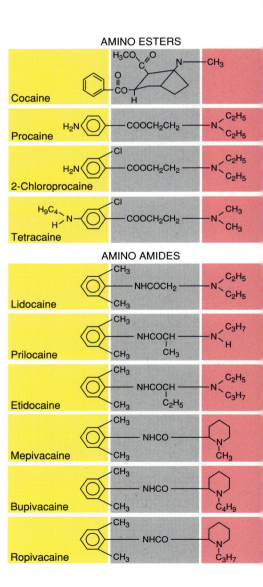

Amino Esters

Cocaine was the first local anesthetic used clinically, and its use today is primarily for topical airway anesthesia. It is unique among the local anesthetics in being a vasoconstrictor rather than a vasodilator. Some anesthesia departments have limited the availability of cocaine because of fears of its abuse potential. In those institutions, mixtures of lidocaine and phenylephrine, rather than cocaine, are utilized to anesthetize airway mucosa and shrink the mucous membranes.

Procaine was synthesized in 1904 by Einhorn, who was looking for a drug that was superior to cocaine and other solutions in use at the turn of the century. Currently, procaine is seldom used for peripheral nerve or epidural blocks because of its low potency, slow onset, short duration of action, and limited power of tissue penetration. It is an excellent local anesthetic for skin infiltration, and its 10% form can be used as a short-acting spinal anesthetic (i.e., less than an hour).

Chloroprocaine has a rapid onset and short duration of action. Its principal use is in performing epidural anesthesia for short cases— i.e., those lasting less than 60 minutes. During the early 1980s its use declined following reports of prolonged sensory and motor deficits that resulted from unintentional subarachnoid administration of an intended epidural dose. Since that time, drug formulation has changed. There is also a question of

back pain developing after large epidural (greater than 30-ml) doses of 3% chloroprocaine.

Tetracaine was first synthesized in 1931, and since that time has become a widely used drug for spinal anesthesia in the United States. It may be used as an isobaric, hypobaric, or hyperbaric solution for spinal anesthesia. Without epinephrine, it typically lasts 1.5 to 2.5 hours, and with the addition of epinephrine may last up to 4 hours for lower extremity procedures. Additionally, tetracaine is an effective topical airway anesthetic, although caution must be used because the potential for systemic side effects is always present. Tetracaine is available as a 1% solution for intrathecal use or as anhydrous crystals that are reconstituted as tetracaine solution by the addition of sterile water immediately prior to use. Tetracaine is not as stable as procaine or lidocaine in solution, and the crystals also undergo deterioration over time. In spite of that caution, when a tetracaine spinal anesthetic is ineffective, one should question technique prior to "blaming" the drug.

Amino Amides

Lidocaine was the first clinically used amide local anesthetic, having been introduced by Lofgren in 1948. Lidocaine has become the most widely used local anesthetic in the world because of its inherent potency, rapid onset, tissue penetration, and effectiveness during infiltration, peripheral nerve block, and both epidural and spinal blocks. During peripheral nerve block, a 1% to 1.5% solution is often effective in producing an acceptable motor blockade, whereas during epidural block a 2% solution seems most effective. When used for spinal anesthesia, a 5% solution in dextrose is its most common form, although it can be used as a short-acting hypobaric solution by utilizing 0.5% lidocaine in a 6- to 8-ml volume. Patients often report lidocaine as causing the most common "local anesthetic allergy." Nevertheless, it should be kept in mind that many of these reported allergies are simply epinephrine reactions from intravascular injection of the local anesthetic epinephrine mixture, often during dental injection.

Prilocaine is structurally related to lidocaine, although it causes significantly less vasodilatation than lidocaine does and thus can be used without epinephrine. Prilocaine is formulated for infiltration, peripheral nerve block, and epidural anesthesia. Its anesthetic profile is similar to that of lidocaine, although, in addition to producing less vasodilatation, it has less potential for systemic toxicity in equal doses. This attribute makes it particularly useful for intravenous regional anesthesia. The major reason prilocaine is not more widely used is that it can result in formation of methemoglobinemia. This results from the metabolism of prilocaine leading to both ortho-toluidine and nitro-toluidine, with both of these capable of causing methemoglobin formation.

Etidocaine is chemically related to lidocaine and is a long-acting amide local anesthetic. Etidocaine is associated with profound motor blockade and is best used when that can be of clinical advantage. It has a more rapid onset of action than bupivacaine has although, compared with bupivacaine, it is infrequently used. Those clinicians using etidocaine often utilize it for the initial epidural dose and then follow subsequent epidural injections with bupivacaine.

Mepivacaine is structurally related to lidocaine, and the two drugs have similar actions. Overall, mepivacaine is slightly longer acting than lidocaine, and this difference in duration is accentuated when epinephrine is added to the solutions.

Bupivacaine is a long-acting local anesthetic that can be used for infiltration, peripheral nerve block, and epidural and spinal anesthesia. Useful concentrations of the drug range from 0.125% to 0.75%. By altering the concentration of bupivacaine, separation of sensory and motor blockade can be achieved. Logically, lower concentrations provide sensory blockade principally, whereas as concentration is increased, effectiveness of motor blockade is increased. If an anesthesiologist had to select a single drug and a single drug concentration, 0.5% bupivacaine would be a logical choice, since at that concentration it is useful for peripheral nerve block, subarachnoid block, and epidural blockade. Interest developed in the 1980s concerning cardiotoxicity during systemic toxic reactions with bupivacaine. Although it is clear that bupivacaine alters myocardial conduction more dramatically than lidocaine does, the need for appropriate and rapid resuscitation during any systemic toxic reaction cannot be overemphasized.

Ropivacaine is another long-acting local anesthetic, similar to bupivacaine, that is being investigated. It is likely to be introduced soon, since it appears to be less cardiotoxic than bupivacaine. It appears to be slightly shorter-acting than bupivacaine, with useful drug concentrations ranging from 0.25% to 1% ropivacaine.

Vasoconstrictors

Vasoconstrictors are often added to local anesthetics to prolong the duration of action and improve the "quality" of the local anesthetic blockade. Although it is still unclear whether vasoconstrictors actually allow local anesthetics to have a longer duration of blockade or are effective because they actually produce additional anti-nociception through alpha-adrenergic action, their clinical effect is not in question. *Epinephrine* (Fig. 1–5) is the most common vasoconstrictor used; overall, the most effective concentration, excluding spinal anesthesia, is a 1:200,000 concentration. When epinephrine is added to local anesthetic in the commercial production process, it is necessary to add stabilizing agents since epinephrine rapidly loses its potency on exposure to air and light. The added stabilizing agents lower the pH of local anesthetic solution into the 3 to 4 range and, because of the higher pKas of local anesthetics, slow the onset of effective regional block. Thus, if epinephrine is to be used with local anesthetics, it should be added at the time the block is performed.

Phenylephrine (Fig. 1–5) also has been used as a vasoconstrictor, principally with spinal anesthesia; effective prolongation of block can be achieved by adding 2 to 5 mg of phenylephrine to the spinal anesthetic drug. Norepinephrine also has been used as a vasoconstrictor for spinal anesthesia, although it does not appear to be as long lasting as, or to have any advantages over, epinephrine. Since most local anesthetics are vasodilators, the addition of epinephrine often does not decrease blood flow as many fear; rather, the combination of local anesthetic and epinephrine results in tissue blood flow similar to that prior to injection.

Needles, Catheters, and Syringes

Effective regional anesthesia requires an anesthesiologist to have comprehensive knowledge both of local anesthetics and of equipment—that is, the needles, syringes, and catheters that allow the anesthetic to be injected into the desired area. In early years, regional anesthesia found many variations in the method of joining needle to syringe.

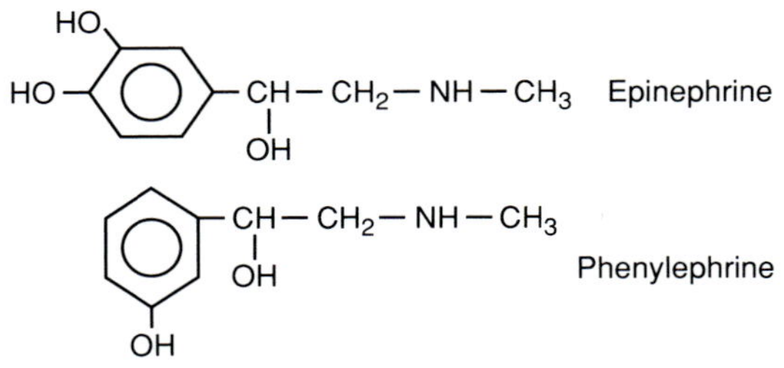

Figure 1–5 Chemical structures of epinephrine and phenylephrine

Around the turn of the century, Carl Schneider developed the first all-glass syringe for Hermann Wolfing-Luer. Luer is credited with the innovation of a simple conical tip for easy exchange of needle to syringe, but the "Luer lock" found in use on most syringes today is thought to have been designed by Dickenson in about 1925. The Luer fitting became virtually universal, and both the Luer slip tip and the Luer-Lok were standardized in 1955.

In almost all disposable and reusable needles used in regional anesthesia, the bevel is cut on three planes. The design theoretically creates less tissue laceration and discomfort than earlier styles did, and it limits tissue coring. Needles that are to be used for deep injection during regional block should incorporate a security bead into their shaft so that the needle is easily retrievable on the rare occasion that needle hub separates from needle shaft. Figure 1–6 contrasts a short, beveled, 22-gauge security bead needle with a 22-gauge "hypodermic" needle. Traditional teaching holds that the short-beveled needle is less traumatic to neural structures. There is little clinical evidence that this is so.

Figure 1–7 is a collage of spinal needles. The key to their successful use is to find the size and bevel tip that allows one to cannulate the subarachnoid space easily without repeated unrecognized puncture. For equivalent needle size, it appears that rounded needle tips that spread the dural fibers are associated with a lesser incidence of headache than are those that cut fibers. The increasing interest in very-small-gauge spinal catheters to reduce the incidence of spinal headache, with controllability of a continuous technique, clearly is going to require additional studies, since the very small caliber of these spinal catheters often seems to complicate spinal anesthesia unduly.

Figure 1–8 depicts epidural needles. Nee-

Figure 1–6 *A–C*, Comparison of short-beveled regional block needle (left in photos) and ''hypodermic'' needle (right in photos)

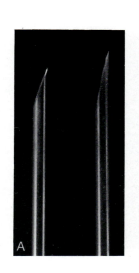
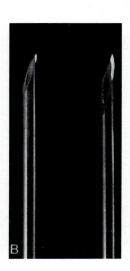
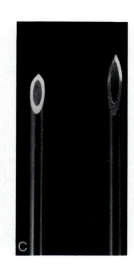

Figure 1–7 Assorted spinal needles. *A, B,* Reusable 22-guage Greene; *C, D,* Disposable 25-gauge Quincke; *E, F,* Reusable 22-gauge Quincke

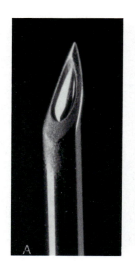
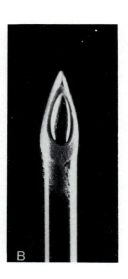

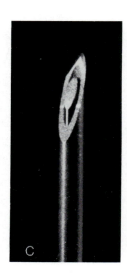
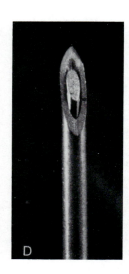
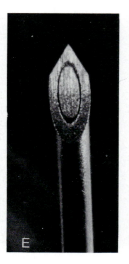
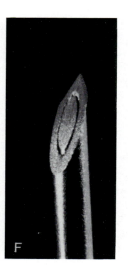

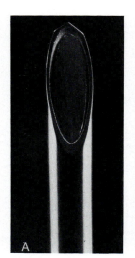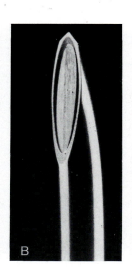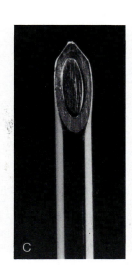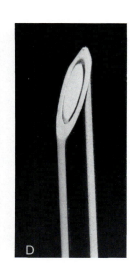

Figure 1—8 Assorted epidural needles. *A*, *B*, Huber; *C*, *D*, reusable Crawford

dle tip design is often mandated by the decision to use a catheter with the epidural technique. Figure 1—9 is a group of the catheters available for either subarachnoid or epidural use. Although each has advantages and disadvantages, a single end-hole catheter appears to provide the highest level of certainty of catheter tip location at the time of injection. Figure 1—10 is a sample of an implantable epidural catheter that can be used for outpatient opioid analgesia, primarily in cancer patients. This is one catheter in which multiple end holes can be utilized successfully, since the catheters are often inserted with fluoroscopic guidance and thus location of the many catheter openings is not an issue.

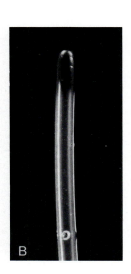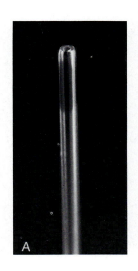

Figure 1—9 Centroneuraxis catheters available for epidural or subarachnoid use. *A*, Single-end hole catheter. *B*, Closed-tip, multiple-sided hole catheter

Nerve Stimulators

It often seems that those recommending the use of nerve stimulators for regional anesthesia do more to impede the successful use of regional anesthesia than they do to advance the techniques. The primary impediment to successfully using a nerve stimulator in a clinical practice is that it becomes at least a three-handed or two-individual technique (Fig. 1—11). Most anesthetic practices do not have the luxury of involving an additional person in performing regional blockade; thus, the idea that a nerve stimulator will somehow allow more "accurate" placement of the regional block needle eventually re-

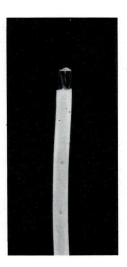

Figure 1—10 Permanent epidural catheter, Silastic implantable

Figure 1–11 Nerve
stimulator technique

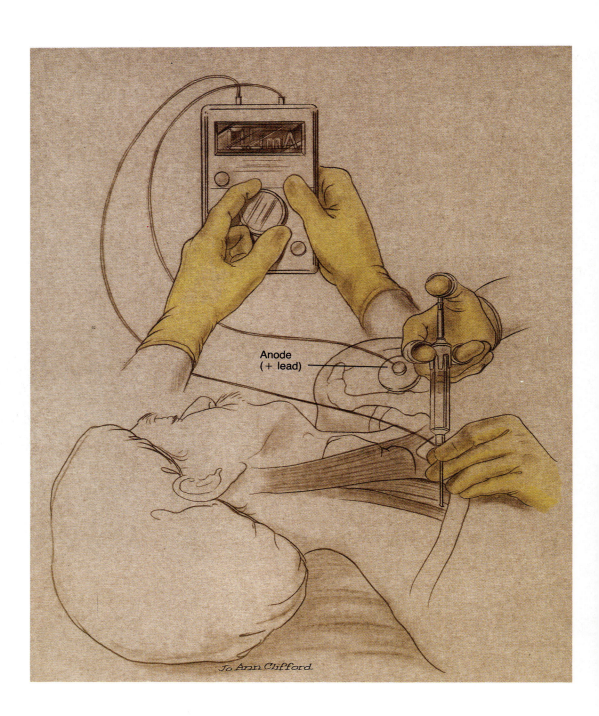

Anode
(+ lead)

Jo Ann Clifford

sults in a decreasing use of regional techniques. Despite this fundamental concern about the use of peripheral nerve stimulators for routine regional blockade, in some circumstances a nerve stimulator can be helpful—e.g., in children and adults who are already anesthetized when a decision is made that regional block is an appropriate technique, or in those individuals who are un-

able to report paresthesias accurately. In addition, another group who may be able to benefit from nerve stimulation are patients with chronic pain, in whom accurate needle placement and reproduction of the pain with electrical stimulation may improve the diagnosis and treatment.

When nerve stimulation is used during regional block, insulated needles are the most appropriate, since the current from such a needle results in a sphere around the needle tip, whereas uninsulated needles emit current at their tip as well as along the shaft, potentially resulting in less precise needle location. A peripheral nerve stimulator should allow between 0.1 and 10 milliamperes of current in pulses lasting approximately 200 milliseconds at a frequency of 1 pulse per second. The peripheral nerve stimulator chosen should also have a digital display of the current delivered with each pulse. This facilitates generalized location of the nerve while stimulating at 2 milliamperes and refinement of needle positioning as the current pulse is reduced to 0.5 to 0.1 milliampere. The nerve stimulator also should have the polarity of the terminals clearly identified, since peripheral nerves are most effectively stimulated by using the needle as the cathode (negative terminal). If the circuit is established with the needle as anode (positive terminal), approximately four times as much current is necessary for stimulation. Thus, the positive lead of the stimulator should be established remote from the site of stimulation by connecting the lead to a common electrocardiographic electrode (Fig. 1–11).

A chief caution in using the nerve stimulator is to approach the nerve block as though the nerve stimulator were not going to be used—that is, as much attention should be paid to the anatomy and technique when using a nerve stimulator as without its use. Only after approaching the block in that manner should the nerve stimulator be utilized for "fine tuning" the block. When the stimulator is used, the current should be adjusted to a level of approximately 2 milliamperes and the needle slowly advanced toward the nerve. If one is stimulating a mixed nerve, muscle stimulation will be observed when the needle is 1 to 2 cm from the nerve. Since large myelinated motor fibers are stimulated by less current than are smaller and unmyelinated fibers, muscle contraction is most often produced prior to patient discomfort. The needle should be repositioned at a point where muscle contraction can be elicited with 0.5 to 0.1 milliampere. If a pure sensory nerve is to be blocked, a similar procedure is followed; however, localization will require the patient to report a sense of pulsed "tingling or burning" over the cutaneous distribution of the sensory nerve. Once the needle is in final position and stimulation is achieved with 0.5 to 0.1 milliampere, 1 ml of local anesthetic should be injected through the needle. If the needle is accurately positioned, this amount of solution should abolish the muscle contraction and/or sensation with pulsed current.

2

Upper Extremity Block Anatomy

*"Man uses his arms and hands constantly . . .
as a result he exposes his arms and hands to injury constantly. . . . Man also eats constantly. . . .
Man's stomach is never really empty. . . . The
combination of man's prehensibility and his un-
flagging appetite keeps a steady flow of patients
with injured upper extremities and full stomachs
streaming into hospital emergency rooms. This is
why the brachial plexus is so frequently the anesthesiologist's favorite group of nerves."*

Classical Anesthesia Files, David Little, 1963

The late David Little's appropriate obser-
vations do not always lead anesthesiologists
to choose a regional anesthetic for upper extremity surgery. However, those who do select regional anesthesia recognize that there
are multiple sites at which the brachial plexus block can be induced. I believe that, if anesthesiologists are to deliver comprehensive
anesthesia care, they should be familiar with
brachial plexus blockade. Familiarity with
these techniques demands that brachial plexus anatomy be understood. One problem
with "understanding" this anatomy is that
the traditional wiring diagram for the brachial plexus is unnecessarily complex and intimidating.

Figure 2–1 illustrates that the plexus is
formed by the ventral rami of the fifth to
eighth cervical nerves and the greater part of
the ramus of the first thoracic nerve. Additionally, small contributions may be made by
the fourth cervical and the second thoracic
nerves. The intimidating part of this anatomy
is what happens from the time these ventral
rami emerge from between the middle and
anterior scalene muscles until they end in the
four terminal branches to the upper extremity: the musculocutaneous, median, ulnar,
and radial nerves. Most of what happens to
the roots on their way to becoming peripheral nerves is not clinically essential information for an anesthesiologist. There are some
broad concepts that may help a clinician's
understanding of brachial plexus anatomy;
throughout, my goal will be to simplify this
anatomy.

After the roots pass between the scalene
muscles, they reorganize into trunks—superi-

or, middle, and inferior. The trunks continue
toward the first rib. At the lateral edge of the
first rib, these trunks undergo a primary anatomic division, into ventral and dorsal divisions. This is also the point at which understanding of brachial plexus anatomy gives
way to frustration and often unnecessary
complexity. This anatomic division is significant because nerves destined to supply the
originally ventral part of the upper extremity
separate from those that supply the dorsal
part. As these divisions enter the axilla, the
divisions give way to cords. The posterior divisions of all three trunks unite to form the

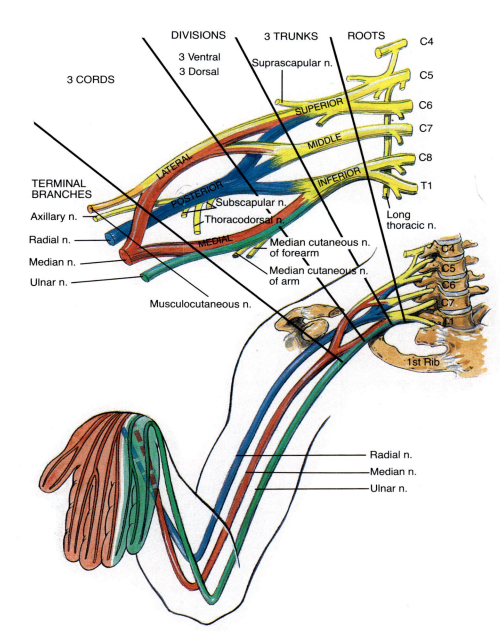

Figure 2–1 Brachial
plexus anatomy

posterior cord; the anterior divisions of the superior and middle trunks form the lateral cord; and the medial cord is the ununited, anterior division of the inferior trunk. These cords are named according to their relationship to the second part of the axillary artery.

At the lateral border of the pectoralis minor muscle, the three cords reorganize to give rise to the peripheral nerves of the upper extremity. Once again, in an effort to simplify, the branches of the lateral and medial cords are all "ventral" nerves to the upper extremity. The posterior cord, in contrast, provides all "dorsal" innervation to the upper extremity. Thus, the radial nerve supplies all the dorsal musculature in the upper extremity below the shoulder. The musculocutaneous nerve supplies muscular innervation in the arm, while providing cutaneous innervation to the forearm. In contrast, the median and ulnar nerves are nerves of passage in the arm, but in the forearm and hand they provide the ventral musculature with motor innervation. These nerves can be further categorized: the median nerve innervates more heavily in the forearm, whereas the ulnar nerve innervates more heavily in the hand.

Some have focused anesthesiologists' attention on the fascial investment of the bra-

Figure 2–2 Upper extremity peripheral nerve innervation with arm supinated on arm board

chial plexus. As the brachial plexus nerve roots leave the transverse processes, they do so between prevertebral fascia that divides to invest both the anterior and middle scalene muscles. Many suggest that this prevertebral fascia surrounding the brachial plexus is tubular in form throughout its course, thus allowing needle placement within the "sheath" to produce brachial plexus blockade easily. There is no question that the brachial plexus is invested with prevertebral fascia; however, it appears that the fascial covering is discontinuous, with septa subdividing portions of the sheath into compartments that clinically may prevent adequate spread of local anesthetics. My clinical impression is that the discontinuity of the "sheath" increases as one moves from transverse process to axilla.

Most upper extremity surgery is performed with the patient resting supine on an operating room table with the arm extended on an arm board. Thus, it seems logical that anesthesiologists clearly understand and picture the innervation of the upper extremity while the patient is in this position. Figures 2–2 through 2–7 illustrate these features with the arm in supinated and pronated positions for cutaneous nerves and dermatomal and osteotomal patterns, respectively.

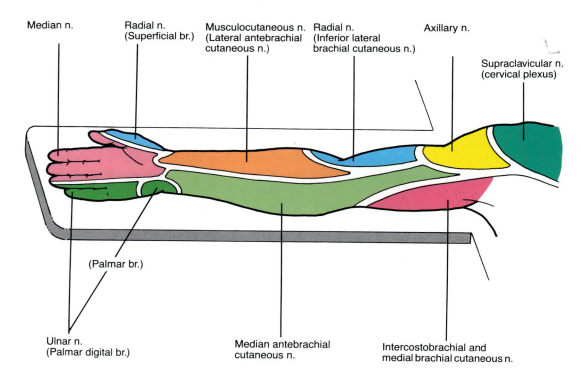

Median n.

Radial n.
(Superficial br.)

Musculocutaneous n.
(Lateral antebrachial
cutaneous n.)

Radial n.
(Inferior lateral
brachial cutaneous n.)

Axillary n.

Supraclavicular n.
(cervical plexus)

(Palmar br.)

Ulnar n.
(Palmar digital br.)

Median antebrachial
cutaneous n.

Intercostobrachial and
medial brachial cutaneous n.

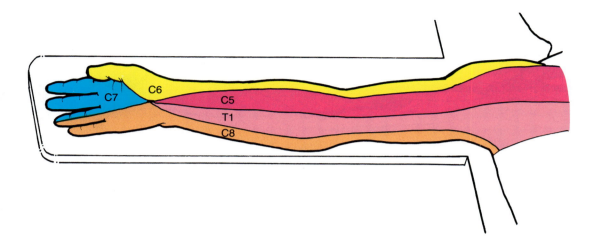

Figure 2–3 Upper extremity dermatome innervation with arm supinated on arm board

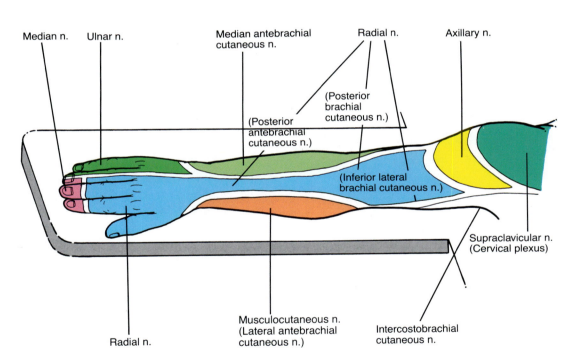

Figure 2–4 Upper extremity peripheral nerve innervation with arm pronated on arm board

Median n.

Ulnar n.

Median antebrachial cutaneous n.

Radial n.

Axillary n.

(Posterior brachial cutaneous n.)

(Posterior antebrachial cutaneous n.)

(Inferior lateral brachial cutaneous n.)

Supraclavicular n. (Cervical plexus)

Musculocutaneous n. (Lateral antebrachial cutaneous n.)

Intercostobrachial cutaneous n.

Radial n.

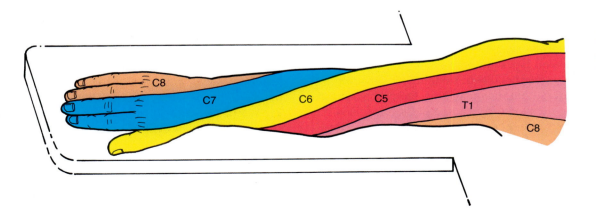

Figure 2–5 Upper extremity dermatome innervation with arm pronated on arm board

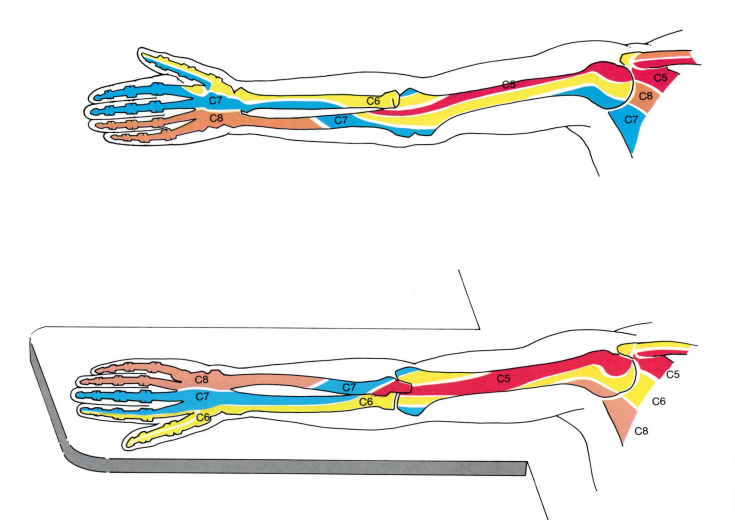

Figure 2–6 Upper extremity osteotomes with arm supinated

Figure 2–7 Upper extremity osteotomes with arm pronated on arm board

An additional clinical "pearl" that will help anesthesiologists in checking brachial plexus blocks prior to the initiation of the surgical procedure is the series of "four Ps." Figure 2–8 illustrates that by using the mnemonic "push, pull, pinch, pinch" an anesthesiologist can remember how to check the four peripheral nerves of interest in brachial plexus blockade. By having the patient resist the anesthesiologist's pulling the forearm away from the upper arm, motor innervation to the biceps muscle can be assessed. If this muscle has been weakened, one can be certain that local anesthetic has reached the musculocutaneous nerve. Likewise, by having the patient attempt to extend the forearm by contracting the triceps muscle, one can as-

sess the radial nerve. Finally, if the patient is pinched in the distribution of the ulnar or median nerve—that is, at the base of the fifth or second digit, respectively—one can develop a sense of the adequacy of block of both the ulnar and median nerves. Typically, if these maneuvers are performed shortly after brachial plexus blockade, motor weakness will be evident prior to sensory block. As a historical highlight, this technique for checking the upper extremity was developed during World War II to allow medics a method of quick analysis of injuries to the brachial plexus.

Some of the brachial plexus neural anatomy of interest to anesthesiologists has been outlined, yet there remain some anatomic

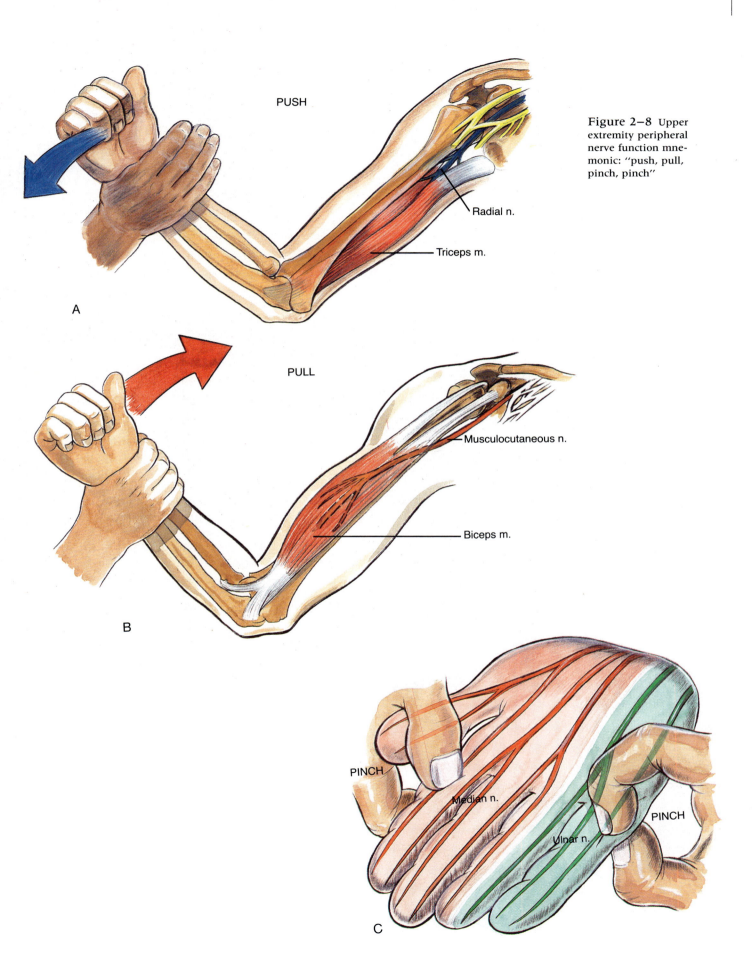

PUSH

Radial n.

Triceps m.

A

PULL

Musculocutaneous n.

Biceps m.

B

PINCH

Median n.

Ulnar n.

PINCH

PINCH

C

Figure 2–8 Upper extremity peripheral nerve function mnemonic: ''push, pull, pinch, pinch''

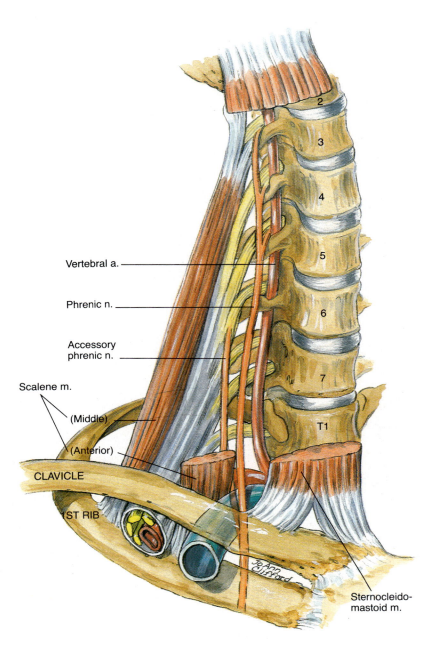

Figure 2–9 "Supra-clavicular" regional block—functional anatomy

details that need to be highlighted (Fig. 2–9). As the cervical roots leave the transverse processes on their way to the brachial plexus, they exit in the gutter in the transverse process immediately posterior to the vertebral artery. The vertebral arteries leave the brachiocephalic and subclavian arteries on the right and left, respectively, and travel cephalad to enter a bony canal in the transverse process at the level of C6 and above. Thus, one must be constantly aware of needle tip location in relationship to the vertebral artery. It should be remembered that the vertebral artery lies anterior to the roots of the brachial plexus as they leave the cervical vertebrae.

Another structure of interest to brachial plexus anatomy is the phrenic nerve. It is formed from branches of the third, fourth, and fifth cervical nerves and passes through the neck on its way to the thorax on the ventral surface of the anterior scalene muscle. It is frequently blocked during interscalene blockade and less frequently with supraclavicular techniques. Avoidance of phrenic blockade is important in only a small percentage of patients, although its location should be kept in mind for those with significantly decreased pulmonary function—that is, those whose day-to-day activities are limited by their pulmonary impairment.

Another detail of brachial plexus anatomy that needs amplification is the organization of the brachial plexus nerves (divisions) as they cross the first rib. Textbooks often depict the nerves in a stacked arrangement at this point. However, radiologic, clinical, and anatomic investigations demonstrate that the nerves are not discretely "stacked" at this point but rather are found in a posterior and cephalic relationship to the subclavian artery (Fig. 2–10). This becomes important when one is carrying out supraclavicular nerve block and using the rib as an anatomic landmark. The relationship of the nerves to the artery means that, if one simply walks the needle tip closely along the first rib, one may not as easily elicit paresthesias, because the nerves are more cephalic in relationship to the first rib.

Labels on figure:
Vertebral a.
Phrenic n.
Accessory phrenic n.
Scalene m.
(Middle)
(Anterior)
CLAVICLE
1ST RIB
Sternocleido-mastoid m.
2
3
4
5
6
7
T1

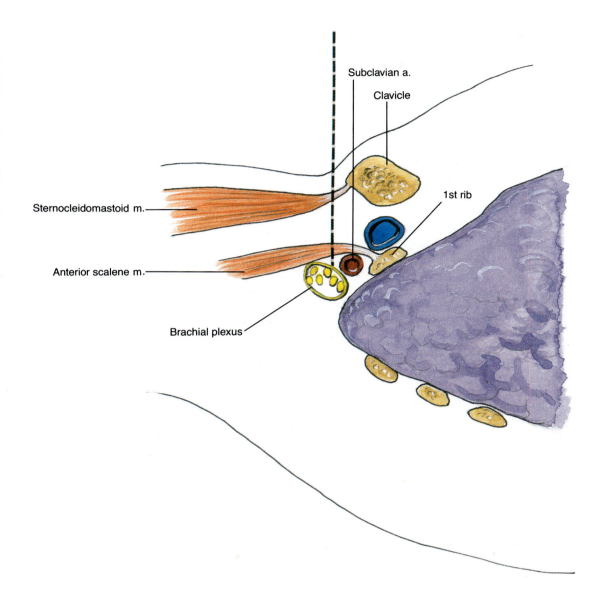

Sternocleidomastoid m.

Anterior scalene m.

Brachial plexus

Subclavian a.

Clavicle

1st rib

Figure 2−10
Supraclavicular block anatomy: functional anatomy of brachial plexus, subclavian artery, and first rib

3

Interscalene Block

Perspective

Interscalene block is especially effective for surgery of the shoulder or upper arm, as the roots of the brachial plexus are most easily blocked with this technique. There is frequently sparing of the ulnar nerve and its more peripheral distribution in the hand, unless one makes a special effort to inject local anesthetic caudad to the site of the initial paresthesia. This block is ideal for reduction of a dislocated shoulder and often can be achieved with as little as 10 to 15 ml of local anesthetic. This block also can be performed with the arm in almost any position and, thus, can be useful when brachial plexus blockade needs to be repeated during a prolonged upper extremity procedure.

Patient Selection. Interscalene blockade is applicable to nearly all patients, since even obese patients usually have identifiable scalene and vertebral body anatomy. However, avoid interscalene blockade in patients with significantly impaired pulmonary function. This point is likely moot if one is planning to use a combined regional and general anesthetic technique, which allows control of ventilation intraoperatively. Even when a long-acting local anesthetic is chosen for the interscalene technique, usually phrenic nerve and thus pulmonary function have returned to a level that patients will tolerate by the time the average length surgical procedure is completed.

Pharmacologic Choice. Useful agents for interscalene blockade are primarily the amino amides. Lidocaine and mepivacaine will produce from 2 to 3 hours of surgical anesthesia without epinephrine and 3 to 5 hours when epinephrine is added. These drugs can be useful for less involved or outpatient surgical procedures. For more extensive surgical procedures requiring hospital admission, a longer-acting agent such as bupivacaine can be chosen. The more complex surgical procedures on the shoulder often require muscle relaxation; thus, bupivacaine concentrations of at least 0.5% are needed. Plain bupivicaine will produce surgical anesthesia lasting from 4 to 6 hours; the addition of epinephrine may prolong this to 8 to 12 hours.

Placement

Anatomy. Surface anatomy of importance to anesthesiologists includes the larynx, sternocleidomastoid muscle, and external jugular vein. Interscalene blockade is most often performed at the level of the C6 vertebral body, which is at the level of the cricoid cartilage. Thus, by projecting a line laterally from the cricoid cartilage, the level at which one should roll the fingers off the sternocleidomastoid muscle onto the belly of the anterior scalene and then into the interscalene groove can be identified. With firm pressure, in most individuals it is possible to feel the transverse process of C6, and in some people it is possible to elicit a paresthesia by deep palpation. The external jugular vein often overlies the interscalene groove at the level of C6, although this should not be relied upon (Fig. 3–1).

It is always important to visualize what lies under the palpating fingers, and, again, the key to carrying out successful interscalene blockade is the identification of the interscalene groove. Figure 3–2 allows us to look beneath surface anatomy and develop a sense of how closely the lateral border of the

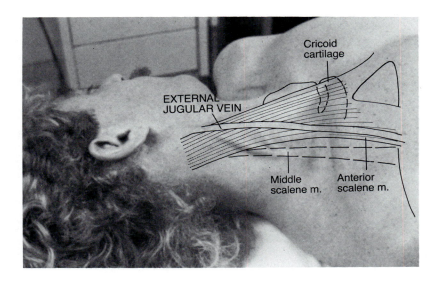

Figure 3–1 Interscalene block—surface anatomy

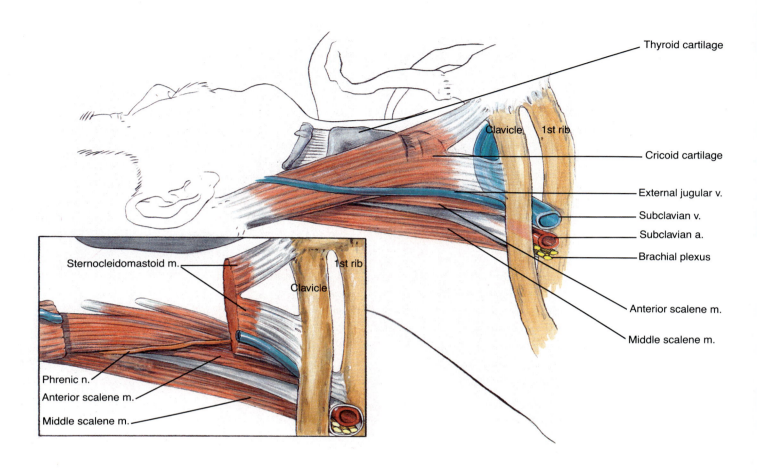

Thyroid cartilage

Clavicle   1st rib

Cricoid cartilage

External jugular v.

Subclavian v.

Subclavian a.

Brachial plexus

Anterior scalene m.

Middle scalene m.

Sternocleidomastoid m.

1st rib

Clavicle

Phrenic n.

Anterior scalene m.

Middle scalene m.

Figure 3–2 Interscalene block—functional anatomy of scalene muscles

anterior scalene muscle parallels the border of the sternocleidomastoid. This feature should be constantly kept in mind. Figure 3–3 removes the anterior scalene and highlights that at the level of C6 the vertebral artery begins its route to the base of the brain by traveling through the root of the transverse process in each of the more cephalad cervical vertebrae.

Position. The patient lies supine with the neck in the neutral position and the head turned slightly opposite the site to be blocked. The anesthesiologist then asks the patient to lift the head off the table to tense the sternocleidomastoid muscle and allow identification of its lateral border. The fingers then roll onto the belly of the anterior scalene and subsequently into the interscalene groove. This maneuver should be carried out in the horizontal plane through the cricoid cartilage, thus, at the level of C6. To roll the fingers effectively (Fig. 3–4), the operator should stand at the patient's side.

Needle Puncture. When the interscalene groove has been identified and the operator's fingers are firmly pressing in the interscalene groove, the needle is inserted, as shown in Figure 3–5, in a slightly caudal and slightly posterior direction. If a paresthesia is not elicited on insertion, the needle is walked, while maintaining the same needle angulation, as shown in Figure 3–4, in a plane joining the cricoid cartilage to the C6 transverse process. Since the brachial plexus is traversing the neck at virtually a right angle to this plane, a paresthesia is almost guaranteed if small enough steps of needle reinsertion are carried out. When undertaking the block for shoulder surgery, this is probably the one brachial plexus block in which a large volume of local anesthetic coupled with a single needle position allows effective anesthesia. For shoulder surgery, 30 to 40 ml of lidocaine, mepivacaine, or bupivacaine can be used. If the interscalene block is being carried out for forearm or hand surgery, a

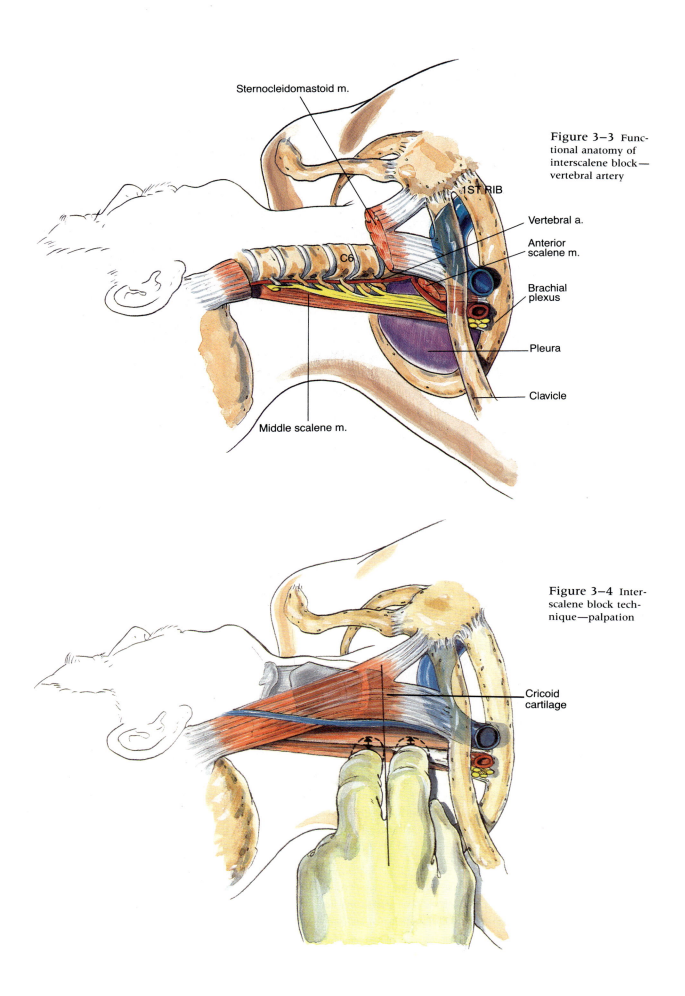

Sternocleidomastoid m.

1ST RIB

C6

Middle scalene m.

Figure 3–3 Functional anatomy of interscalene block—vertebral artery

Vertebral a.

Anterior scalene m.

Brachial plexus

Pleura

Clavicle

Figure 3–4 Interscalene block technique—palpation

Cricoid cartilage

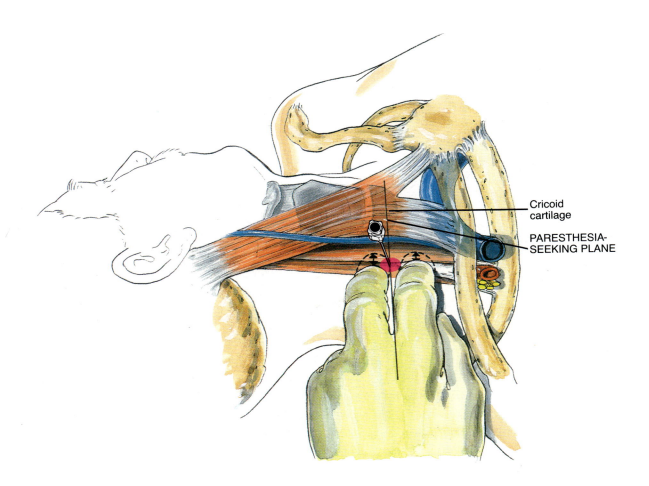

Cricoid
cartilage

PARESTHESIA-
SEEKING PLANE

Figure 3–5 Interscalene block technique—"paresthesia-seeking" plane

second, more caudal needle position is desirable, in which 10 to 20 ml more of local anesthetic is injected to allow spread along more caudal roots.

Potential Problems. Problems that can arise from interscalene blockade include subarachnoid injection, epidural blockade, intravascular injection (especially in the vertebral artery), pneumothorax, and phrenic block.

Pearls

This block is most applicable to shoulder work, in contrast to forearm and hand surgical procedures. When undertaking a block for shoulder surgery that requires muscle relaxation, choose a local anesthetic concentration that provides adequate motor block—that is, mepivacaine and lidocaine at 1.5% concentration and bupivacaine at 0.5% concentration. Since this block is most often carried out through the use of a single injection site and the operator relies on spread of local anesthet-

ic solution, one must allow sufficient "soak time" after the injection. This often means from 20 to 35 minutes.

If there is difficulty identifying the anterior scalene muscle, one maneuver is to have the patient maximally inhale while the anesthesiologist palpates the neck. During this maneuver the scalene muscles should contract before the sternocleidomastoid muscle contracts, and this may allow clarification of the anterior scalene muscle in the difficult-to-palpate neck. Most of the injection difficulties that result in complications of the block can be avoided if one remembers that this should be a very "superficial" block; if the palpating fingers apply sufficient pressure, no more than 1 to 1.5 cm of the needle should be necessary to reach the plexus and a paresthesia. It is when the needle is inserted deeply that one must be cautious about subarachnoid, epidural, and intravascular injection. If one is planning to use the interscalene block for an operation that requires ulnar nerve blockade, I emphasize that this would not be my choice of brachial plexus block. The ulnar nerve is difficult to block with the interscalene approach, since it is derived from the eighth cervical nerve (this nerve is difficult to block following injection at a more cephalic injection site). Finally, one should be cautious about using this block in a patient with significant pulmonary impairment, since phrenic blockade is almost guaranteed with the block.

4

Supraclavicular Block

Perspective

Supraclavicular block will provide anesthesia of the entire upper extremity in the most consistent, time-efficient manner of any brachial plexus technique. It is the most effective block for all portions of the upper extremity and is carried out at the "division" level of the brachial plexus. Perhaps this is why there is often little or no sparing of peripheral nerves if an "adequate" paresthesia is obtained. If this block is to be utilized for shoulder surgery, it should be supplemented with a superficial cervical plexus block to anesthetize skin overlying the shoulder.

Patient Selection. Almost all patients are candidates for this block, with the exception of those who are uncooperative. In addition, in less experienced hands it may be inappropriate for outpatients. Although pneumothorax is an infrequent complication of the block, one often becomes apparent only after a delay of several hours, when an outpatient might already be at home. Also, since the supraclavicular block relies principally on bony and muscular landmarks, very obese patients are not good candidates, because they often have supraclavicular fat pads that interfere with easy application of this technique.

Pharmacologic Choice. As with other brachial plexus blocks, the prime consideration of drug selection should be the length of the procedure and the degree of motor blockade desired. Mepivacaine (1 to 1.5%), lidocaine (1 to 1.5%), and bupivacaine (0.5%) are all applicable to brachial plexus blockade. Lidocaine and mepivacaine will produce from 2 to 3 hours of surgical anesthesia without epinephrine and 3 to 5 hours when epinephrine is added. These drugs can be useful for less involved or outpatient surgical procedures. For extensive surgical procedures requiring hospital admission, a longer-acting agent like bupivacaine can be chosen. Plain bupivacaine will produce surgical anesthesia lasting from 4 to 6 hours, whereas the addition of epinephrine may prolong this to 8 to 12 hours.

Placement

Anatomy. The anatomy of interest for this block is the relationship between brachial plexus and the first rib, subclavian artery, and cupula of the lung (Fig. 4–1). My experience suggests that this block is more difficult to teach than many of the other regional blocks, and for that reason two approaches to the supraclavicular block are illustrated: the classic Kulenkampff approach and the "plumb bob" approach. The plumb bob approach has been developed in an attempt to overcome the difficulty and time necessary to become skilled in the classic supraclavicular block approach. In spite of that caution, either of the techniques is clinically useful, once mastered. As the subclavian artery and brachial plexus pass over the first rib, they do so between insertion of the anterior and middle scalene muscles onto the first rib (Fig. 4–2). The nerves lie in a cephaloposterior relationship to the artery; thus paresthesia may be elicited prior to the needle's contacting the first rib. At the point where the artery and plexus cross the first rib, the first rib is broad and flat, sloping in a caudal direction as it moves from posterior to anterior; and, although the rib is a curved structure, there is a distance of 1 to 2 cm upon which a needle can be walked in an anterior-posterior direction. Remember that immediately medial to this first rib is the cupula of the lung; when the needle angle is too medial, pneumothorax may result.

Position—Classic Supraclavicular Block. The patient lies supine without a pillow, with the head turned opposite to the side to be blocked. The arms are at the sides, and the anesthesiologist can stand either at the head of the table or at the side of the patient, near the arm to be blocked.

Needle Puncture—Classic. In the classic approach, the needle insertion site is approximately 1 cm superior to the clavicle at the clavicular midpoint (Fig. 4–3). It is emphasized that this entry site is closer to the middle of the clavicle than to the junction of the middle and medial third, as often described in other regional texts. Additionally, if the artery is palpable in the supraclavicular fossa, it can be used as a landmark. From this point, the needle and syringe are inserted in a plane approximately parallel to the patient's neck and head, with care taken that the axis of syringe and needle does not aim medially toward the cupula of the lung. The needle should be a 22-gauge, 5-cm needle that typically will contact rib at a depth of 3

Figure 4–1 Supraclavicular block anatomy

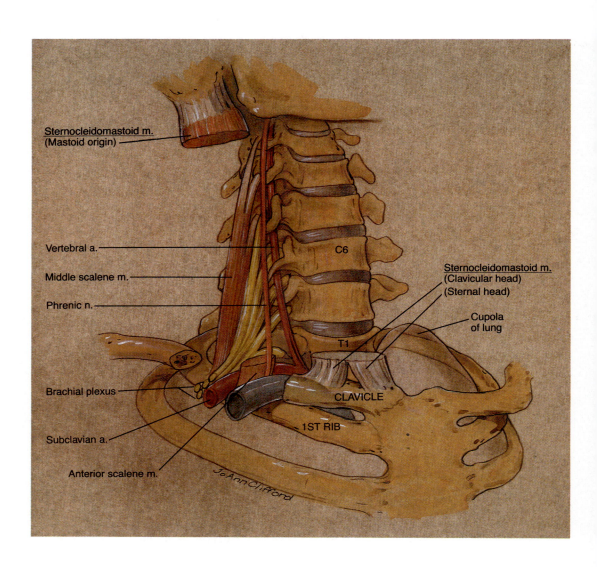

Sternocleidomastoid m. (Mastoid origin)

Vertebral a.

Middle scalene m.

Phrenic n.

Brachial plexus

Subclavian a.

Anterior scalene m.

C6

Sternocleidomastoid m. (Clavicular head) (Sternal head)

Cupola of lung

T1

CLAVICLE

1ST RIB

JoAnn Clifford

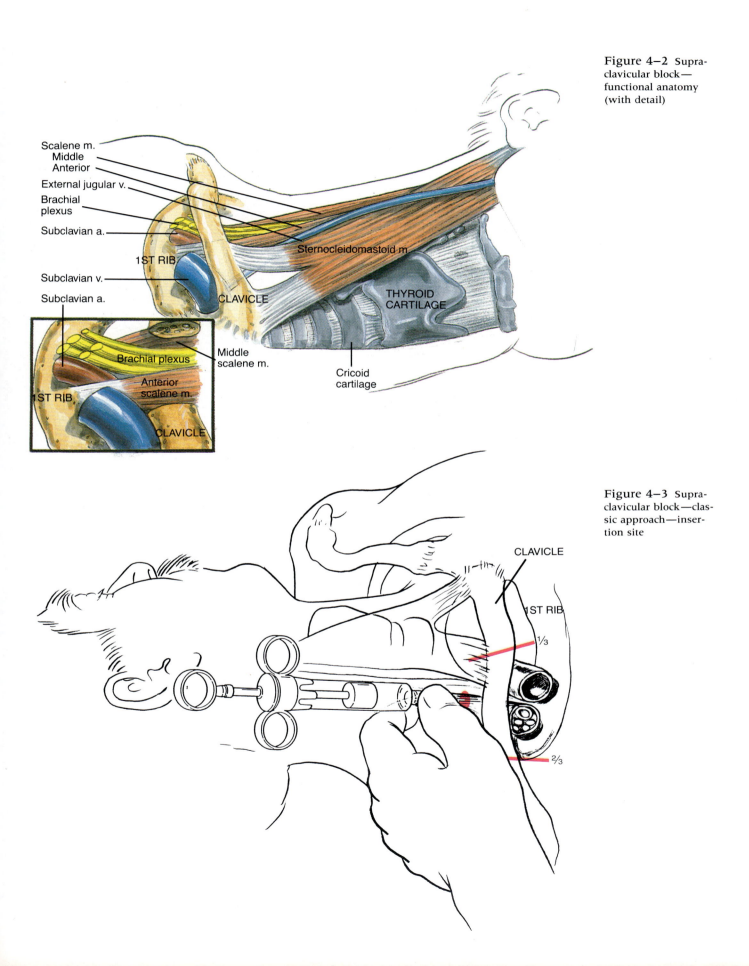

Figure 4–2 Supraclavicular block—functional anatomy (with detail)

Scalene m.
Middle
Anterior
External jugular v.
Brachial plexus
Subclavian a.
1ST RIB
Subclavian v.
Subclavian a.
Brachial plexus
Middle scalene m.
Anterior scalene m.
1ST RIB
CLAVICLE
CLAVICLE
Sternocleidomastoid m
THYROID CARTILAGE
Cricoid cartilage

Figure 4–3 Supraclavicular block—classic approach—insertion site

CLAVICLE
1ST RIB
1/3
2/3

Figure 4–4 Supra-clavicular block—classic approach—hand and syringe assembly positioning

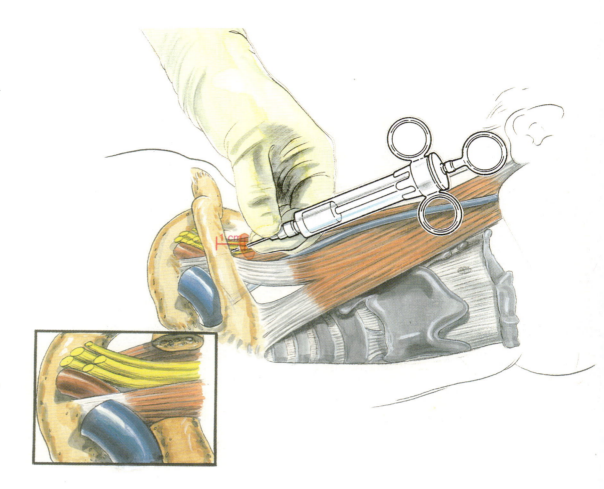

to 4 cm, although it is sometimes necessary to insert to a depth of 6 cm in a very large patient. The initial needle insertion should not be carried out past 3 to 4 cm until a careful search in an anteroposterior plane does not identify the first rib. During the insertion of the needle and syringe, the assembly should be controlled with the hand, as illustrated in Figure 4–4. The hand can rest lightly against the patient's supraclavicular fossa, since with elicitation of a paresthesia patients often move their shoulder.

Position—Plumb Bob Supraclavicular Block. The development of the plumb bob approach of supraclavicular block resulted from efforts to simplify the anatomic projection necessary for the block. The patient should be positioned in a manner similar to that for the classic approach, lying supine without a pillow, with the head turned slightly away from the side to be blocked. The anesthesiologist should stand lateral to the patient at the level of the patient's upper arm. This block involves inserting the needle and syringe assembly at approximately a 90° angle to the classic approach.

Needle Puncture—Plumb Bob. Patients are asked to raise the head slightly off the block table so that the lateral border of the sterno-cleidomastoid muscle can be marked as it inserts onto the clavicle. From that point, a "mental" plane is visualized that runs para-sagittally through that site (Fig. 4–5). The name "plumb bob" was chosen for this block concept since, if one suspends a plumb bob over the entry site as shown in Figure 4–6, needle insertion through that point will result in contact with the brachial plexus in most patients. Figure 4–6 also illustrates a parasagittal section obtained by magnetic resonance scanning in the sagittal plane necessary to carry out this block. As illustrated, the brachial plexus at the level of the first ribs lies posterior and cephalic to the subclavian artery. Once this skin mark has been placed immediately superior to the clavicle at the lateral border of the sternocleidomastoid muscle as it inserts into the clavicle, the needle is inserted in the parasagittal plane at a 90° angle to the table top. If paresthesia is not elicited on the first pass, the needle and syringe are redirected cephalad in small steps

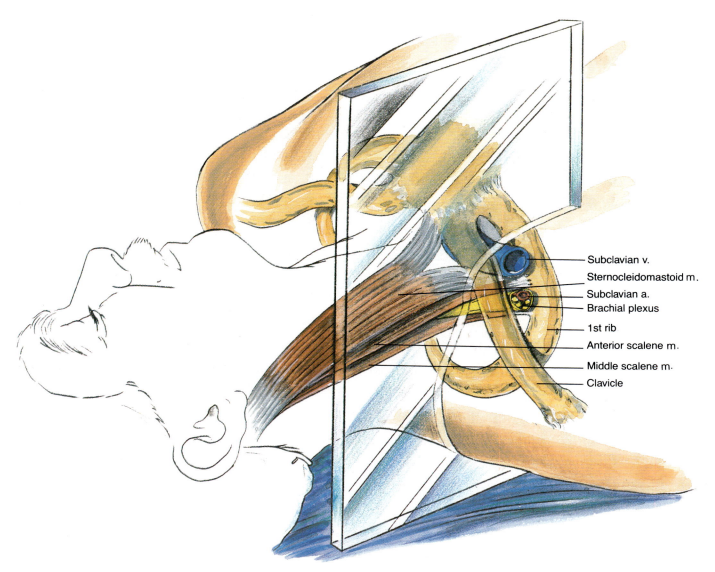

Subclavian v.
Sternocleidomastoid m.
Subclavian a.
Brachial plexus
1st rib
Anterior scalene m.
Middle scalene m.
Clavicle

Figure 4—5 Supra-clavicular block—plumb bob—functional anatomy

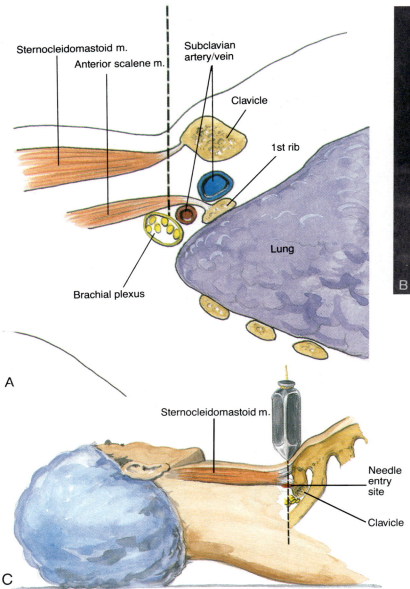

Sternocleidomastoid m.

Anterior scalene m.

Subclavian artery/vein

Clavicle

1st rib

Lung

Brachial plexus

A

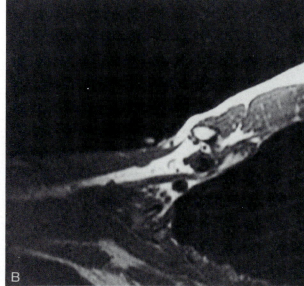

B

Sternocleidomastoid m.

Needle entry site

Clavicle

C

Figure 4–6 Supra-clavicular block—plumb bob—parasagittal magnetic resonance image anatomy

through an arc of approximately 20°. If a paresthesia still has not been obtained, needle and syringe are reinserted at the starting position and then moved in small steps through an arc of approximately 20° in a caudal direction (Fig. 4–7).

Since the brachial plexus lies cephaloposterior to the artery as it crosses the first rib, often a paresthesia can be elicited prior to contacting either the artery or the first rib. If that occurs, approximately 30 ml of local anesthetic is inserted at this single site.

If a paresthesia is not elicited with the maneuvers described but the first rib is contacted, the block is carried out just like the classic approach—walking along the first rib until paresthesia is elicited. Like the classic approach, care should be taken not to allow the syringe and needle assembly to aim medially toward the cupula of the lung.

Potential Problems. The most feared complication of this block is pneumothorax. The principal cause of this is needle/syringe angles that ''aim'' toward the cupula of the

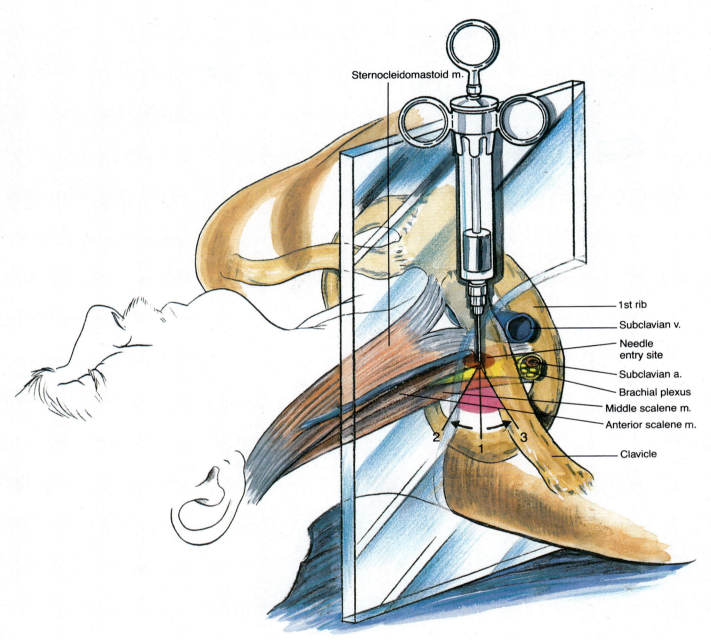

Sternocleidomastoid m.

1st rib

Subclavian v.

Needle
entry site

Subclavian a.

Brachial plexus

Middle scalene m.

Anterior scalene m.

Clavicle

2   1   3

Figure 4–7 Supra-
clavicular block—
plumb bob—paresthe-
sia-seeking approach

lung. Special attention should be directed toward walking the needle in a strict anteroposterior direction. Pneumothorax incidence is between half and 5% and is at the lower end of that range when an anesthesiologist becomes skilled. The cupula of the lung rises proportionally higher in the neck in thin, asthenic individuals, and perhaps in these individuals the incidence of pneumothorax is higher. Development of pneumothorax most often takes a number of hours, thus it is likely related to impingement of the needle upon the lung with subsequent development of pneumothorax, rather than air entering the pleural space as the needle is inserted. Once again, phrenic nerve blockade does occur, probably in the range of 30% to 50%, and the block's use in patients with significantly impaired pulmonary function must be weighed. The development of hematoma following supraclavicular block, as a result of puncture of the subclavian artery, usually simply requires observation.

Pearls

The predictability and rapid onset of this block allow one to "keep up" with even a fast orthopedic surgeon. This is an advantage, since regional anesthesia can be used for hand surgery, even in a busy practice. As previously outlined, this block seems to require a longer time to proficiency than most other regional blocks, and for that reason, the anesthesiologist should develop a system for its use. "Wishful" probing at the root of the neck without a system is not the way to approach this block. Likewise, one should choose either the classic or plumb bob approach and give each a fair trial prior to abandoning either.

If a pneumothorax does occur following supraclavicular block, it most often can be observed while the patient is reassured. If the pneumothorax is large enough to cause dyspnea or patient discomfort, aspiration of the pneumothorax through a small-gauge catheter is often all that is necessary for treatment. The patient should be admitted for observation; however, it is the exceptional patient who needs formal, large-bore chest tube placement for re-expansion of the lung. Obviously difficult patients should not be chosen as one develops expertise with this block.

5

Axillary Block

Perspective

Axillary brachial plexus block is most effective for surgical procedures distal to the elbow. In some patients procedures on the elbow or lower humerus can be carried out with an axillary technique, but strong consideration should be given to supraclavicular block for those more proximal procedures. It is discouraging to carry out a "successful" axillary block only to find that the surgical procedure extends outside the area of blockade. The block is appropriate for hand and forearm surgery; thus it is often the most appropriate technique for outpatients in a busy hand surgery practice. Because this block is carried out distant from both the centroneuraxis and the lung, complications attendant to those areas are avoided.

Patient Selection. For axillary block to be performed, patients must be able to abduct their arm at the shoulder. As experience of the operator increases, the necessity for this diminishes, but this block cannot be carried out with the arm at the side. Since the block is most appropriate for forearm and hand surgery, it is a rare patient with a surgical condition at those sites who cannot abduct the arm as described.

Pharmacologic Choice. Since hand and wrist procedures often require less motor blockade than do those on the shoulder, the concentration of local anesthetic chosen can usually be slightly decreased with axillary block, in contrast to supraclavicular or interscalene block. Appropriate drugs are lidocaine (1 to 1.5%), mepivacaine (1 to 1.5%), and bupivacaine (0.5%). Lidocaine and mepivacaine will produce from 2 to 3 hours of surgical anesthesia without epinephrine and 3 to 5 hours when epinephrine is added. These drugs can be useful for less involved or outpatient surgical procedures. For more extensive surgical procedures requiring hospital admission, a longer-acting agent such as bupivacaine can be chosen. Plain bupivacaine will produce surgical anesthesia lasting from 4 to 6 hours; the addition of epinephrine may prolong this to 8 to 12 hours. The local anesthetic time line must be considered when prescribing a drug for outpatient axillary block, since blocks lasting as long as 18 to 24 hours can result from higher concentrations of bupivacaine with added epinephrine.

Placement

Anatomy. At the level of the distal axilla, where axillary block is undertaken (Fig. 5–1), the axillary artery can be thought of as indicating the center of a four-quadrant neurovascular bundle. It is useful for me to conceptualize these nerves in a quadrant (or clock face) manner, since multiple injections during axillary blockade result in more acceptable clinical anesthesia in my practice than does injection at a single site. The musculocutaneous nerve is found in the 9 to 12 quadrant in the substance of the coracobrachialis muscle. The median nerve is most often in the 12 to 3 quadrant; the ulnar nerve is "inferior" to the median nerve in the 3 to 6 quadrant; and the radial nerve is in the 6 to 9 quadrant. The block does not need to be performed in the axilla and, in fact, needle insertion in the mid to lower portion of the axillary hair patch or even more distal is effective. It is clear from radiographic and anatomic study of the brachial plexus and the axilla that separate and distinct sheaths are associated with the plexus at this point. If this concept is kept in mind, it will help decrease the number of unacceptable blocks.

Position. The patient is placed supine, with the arm forming a 90° angle with the trunk, and the forearm forming a 90° angle with the upper arm (Fig. 5–2). This allows the anesthesiologist to stand at the level of the patient's upper arm and palpate the axillary artery, as illustrated in Figure 5–2. A line should be drawn tracing the course of the artery from the midaxilla to the lower axilla; and overlying this line the index and third fingers of the left hand of the anesthesiologist are used to identify the artery and minimize the amount of subcutaneous tissue overlying the neurovascular bundle. In this manner, the anesthesiologist can develop a sense of the longitudinal course of the artery, which is essential for axillary blockade.

Needle Puncture. While the axillary artery is identified with two fingers, the needle and syringe are inserted as shown in Figure 5–3. It is emphasized that some local anesthetic should be deposited in each of the quadrants surrounding the axillary artery. If paresthesia is obtained, that is beneficial, although undue expenditure of time and patient discomfort should not occur during attempts to elicit

Figure 5–1 Axillary block—functional "quadrant" anatomy of distal axilla

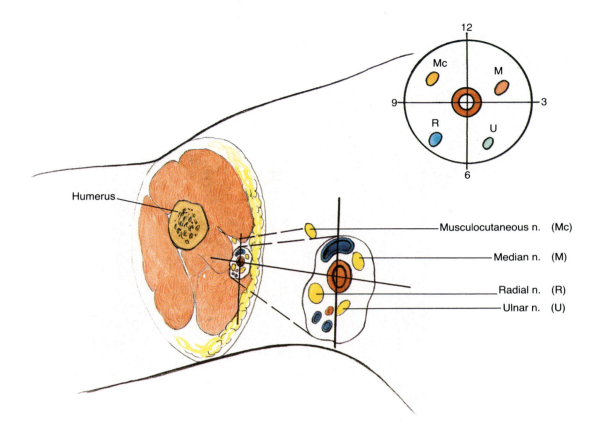

Humerus

Musculocutaneous n.   (Mc)

Median n.   (M)

Radial n.   (R)

Ulnar n.   (U)

Figure 5–2 Axillary block positioning— patient arm and palpating fingers

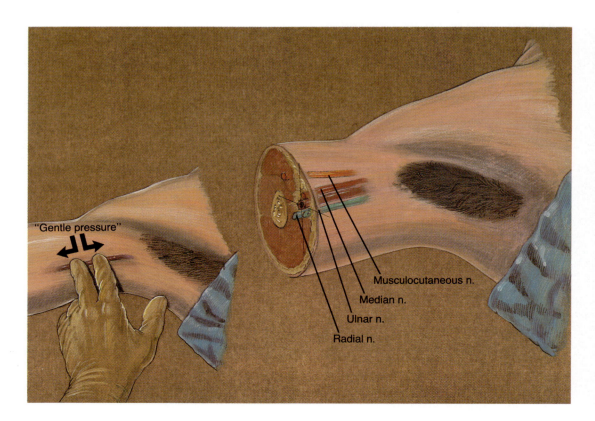

"Gentle pressure"

Musculocutaneous n.

Median n.

Ulnar n.

Radial n.

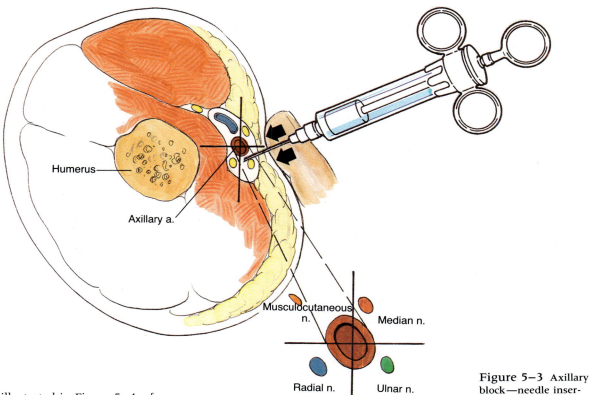

Musculocutaneous
n.

Median n.

Radial n.   Ulnar n.

Humerus

Axillary a.

Figure 5—3 Axillary
block—needle inser-
tion

a paresthesia. As illustrated in Figure 5—4, effective axillary blockade is produced by utilizing the axillary artery as an anatomic landmark and infiltrating in a fanlike manner
around the artery. Anesthesia of the musculocutaneous nerve is best achieved by infiltrating into the mass of the coracobrachial is
muscle. This can be carried out by identifying
the coracobrachial is and injecting into its
substance, or by inserting a longer needle
until it contacts the humerus and injecting in
a fanlike manner (Fig. 5—4).

Potential Problems. Problems with axillary
blockade are infrequent due to the distance
from centroneuraxis structures and the lung.
One complication that can be avoided by the
use of multiple injections rather than using a
fixed needle is the occasional occurrence of
systemic toxicity from axillary block. Any
time a single, immobile needle is used to inject large volumes of a local anesthetic, the
potential for systemic toxicity increases, especially when contrasted with using smaller
volumes of local anesthetic injected at multiple sites. Another potential problem with axillary blockade is development of postopera-

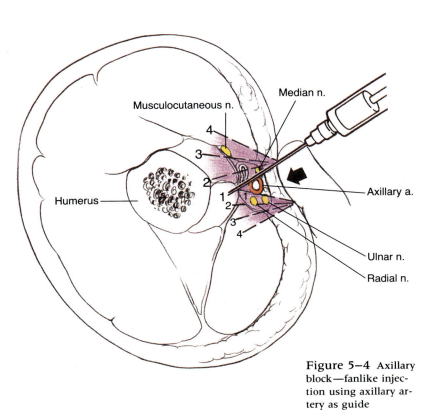

Musculocutaneous n.

Median n.

Humerus

Axillary a.

Ulnar n.

Radial n.

Figure 5—4 Axillary
block—fanlike injec-
tion using axillary ar-
tery as guide

tive neuropathy; one should not assume that axillary blockade is the cause of all neuropathy following upper extremity surgery. A logical and systematic approach to determine the etiology of a neuropathy must be carried out if we are to understand the true incidence and causes of neuropathy following brachial plexus blockade.

Pearls

For axillary blockade to be as effective as possible, one must understand the organization of the peripheral nerves at the level of the lower axilla. It is clear that the axillary sheath at this level is discontinuous and may demand multiple injections to allow the axillary blockade to be effec-

tive. This does not mean that a single injection cannot produce acceptable surgical anesthesia; however, the most consistently effective axillary blockade results from depositing smaller amounts of local anesthetic in multiple sites. Additionally, unnecessarily seeking paresthesia for an extended time, which results in anesthetic delays and patient discomfort, will discourage anesthesiologists from carrying out this block. If one keeps in mind the quadrant approach to axillary blockade, this block should be accomplished in a time-efficient manner. A mnemonic to help is "M&Ms are tops" (i.e., median and musculocutaneous nerves are more cephalic in the abducted arm). Almost everyone is able to relate the "topnotch" candy M&Ms to the cephalic position of the two "m" nerves.

6

Distal Upper Extremity Blocks

Ulnar, Median, and Radial Block at the Elbow

Perspective

In general, distal upper extremity blocks, those at the elbow or wrist, cannot be strongly encouraged. Although definitive data are lacking, the reason is a perception that these more distal peripheral blocks are associated with a slightly higher likelihood of nerve injury, perhaps because many of the peripheral branches are anatomically located in sites where the nerve is contained within bony and ligamentous surroundings. It is not difficult to localize the nerves at these peripheral sites, although the "entrapment" of these nerves makes more proximal blockade, such as the axillary block, my preferred approach. Further, since a significant portion of hand and forearm surgery is carried out using an upper arm tourniquet, purposeful use of more distal blocks mandates significantly heavier sedation so that the patient may tolerate tourniquet inflation pressures.

Patient Selection. Few patients should require distal upper extremity block, although there may be some, such as those needing supplementation following brachial plexus block. In any event, these patients should be few in number, and comprehensive anesthesia care should be possible without frequently utilizing these blocks.

Pharmacologic Choice. These peripheral blocks are usually considered for superficial surgery; thus, lower concentrations of local anesthetic are appropriate since motor blockade should not be an issue. Therefore, 0.75% to 1% mepivacaine or lidocaine, or 0.25% bupivacaine, should be sufficient.

Placement

At the Elbow

Anatomy. Of the three major nerves at the elbow—radial, median, and ulnar—the ulnar is most predictable in location. As illustrated in Figure 6–1, the ulnar nerve is located in the ulnar groove, which is a bony fascial canal between the medial epicondyle of the humerus and the olecranon process. This area is extremely well protected by fibrous tissue and, in spite of what would seem like an easy site to carry out block, the nerve is quite well protected (and potentially vulnerable) in the ulnar groove. The median nerve

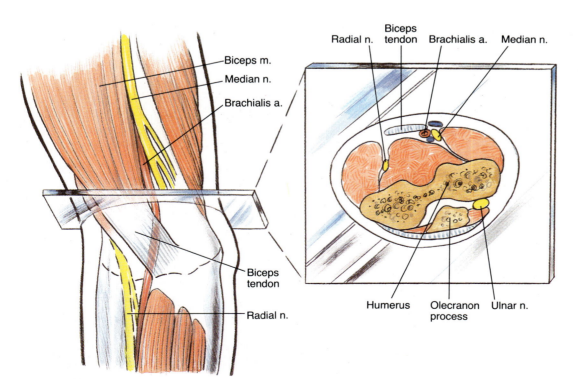

Biceps m.
Median n.
Brachialis a.
Biceps tendon
Radial n.

Radial n.   Biceps tendon   Brachialis a.   Median n.

Humerus   Olecranon process   Ulnar n.

Figure 6–1 Elbow blocks—functional anatomy

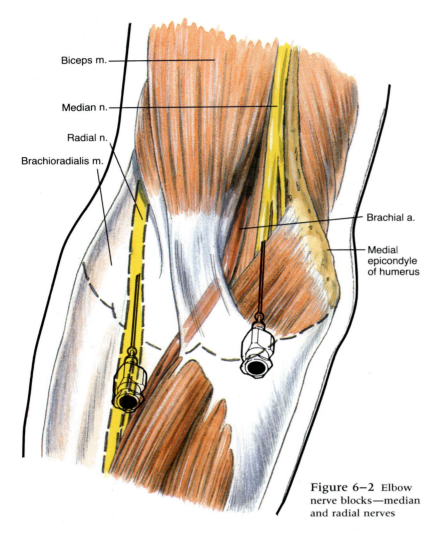

Figure 6–2 Elbow nerve blocks—median and radial nerves

at the elbow lies medial to the brachial artery, which lies just medial to the biceps muscle. Conversely, the radial nerve has a somewhat variable course, pierces the lateral intramuscular septum on its way to the forearm, and lies between the brachialis muscle and the brachioradialis muscle in the distal aspect of the upper arm. It is more effectively blocked in the axilla than at the elbow.

Position. All three of these nerves are blocked with the patient in the supine position and the arm supinated and abducted at the shoulder at a 90° angle. Additionally, when the ulnar nerve block is performed, the forearm is flexed upon the upper arm to identify more easily the ulnar groove (as illustrated in Figure 6–3).

Needle Puncture—Median Nerve Block (Fig. 6–2). A line should be drawn between the medial and lateral epicondyles of the humerus (at the level of the pane of glass shown in Figure 6–1). Immediately medial to the brachial artery, the needle is inserted in the plane of the "pane of glass," and a paresthesia is sought. If no paresthesia is obtained, the injection of 3 to 5 ml of solution medial to the brachial artery should result in median nerve block. If a paresthesia is obtained, a similar amount is injected at that site.

Needle Puncture—Radial Nerve Block (Fig. 6–2). The radial nerve is likewise blocked at the level of the pane of glass in Figure 6–1. The biceps tendon at that level should be identified, and then a mark is made 1 to 2 cm to the tendon. Again, a small-gauge, 3-cm needle is inserted through the mark in the plane of the pane of glass and paresthesia sought. If no paresthesia is obtained, a fanlike injection of 4 to 6 ml of solution is made at that site.

Needle Puncture—Ulnar Nerve Block. As illustrated in Figure 6–3, the forearm is flexed upon the upper arm, and the ulnar groove is palpated. At a point approximately 1 cm proximal to a line drawn between the olecranon process and the medial epicondyle, a needle is inserted. A paresthesia should be easily obtainable, and once it is, the needle is withdrawn a millimeter and 3 to 5 ml of local anesthetic is injected through a small-gauge, 2-cm needle. A larger volume of solution should not be injected directly into the ulnar groove, since high pressure in this tightly contained fascial space may increase the risk of nerve injury.

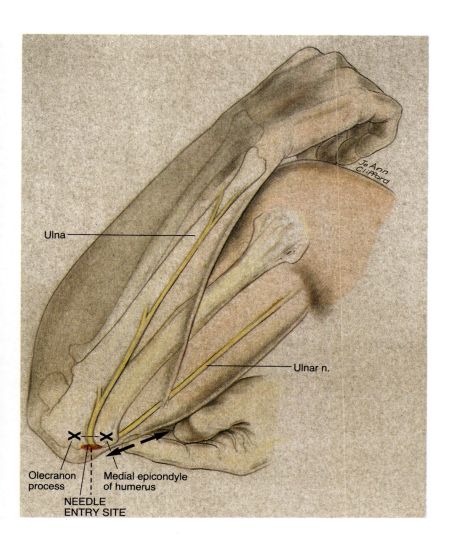

Ulna

Ulnar n.

Olecranon
process

Medial epicondyle
of humerus

NEEDLE
ENTRY SITE

Figure 6–3 Ulnar
nerve block—posi-
tioning

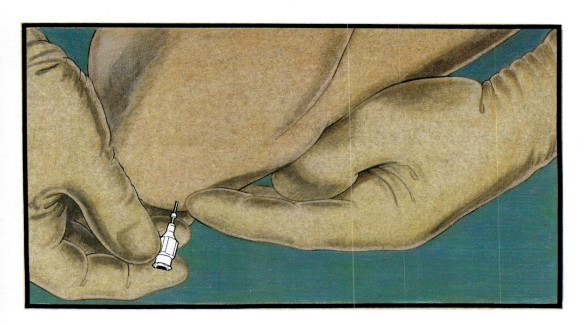

Placement

At the Wrist

Anatomy (Fig. 6–4). The ulnar nerve lies immediately lateral to the tendon of the flexor carpi ulnaris muscle and immediately medial to the ulnar artery. The median nerve lies between the tendon of palmaris longus and the tendon of the flexor carpi radialis muscle. That places the median nerve in the long axis of the radius. The radial nerve at the wrist has already divided into a number of its peripheral branches, and effective blockade requires a field block along the radial aspect of the wrist.

Position (Fig. 6–5). To perform peripheral block at the wrist, the patient rests supine while the arm is extended at the shoulder and supported on an arm board. The wrist is flexed over a small support, and the most effective position for the anesthesiologist is to stand in the long axis of the arm board. Then, while performing the block, the anes-

thesiologist may observe the patient's face during elicitation of paresthesia.

Needle Puncture—Ulnar Nerve Block. Immediately proximal to the ulnar styloid process, it should be easy to palpate the tendon of the flexor carpi ulnaris and the ulnar artery. A small-gauge, short-bevel needle can be inserted perpendicular to the wrist at this site, and a paresthesia should be easy to elicit. Three to five milliliters of solution can be injected at this site; if no paresthesia is obtained, a similar amount can be injected in a fanlike manner between those two structures with near certainty of blockade.

Needle Puncture—Median Nerve Block. On a line between the styloid process of the ulna and the prominence of the distal radius, the palmaris longus tendon and the tendon of the flexor carpi radialis are identified. These tendons can be accentuated by having patients flex the wrists while making a fist. The median nerve lies deep and between those structures, so a blunt-beveled, small-gauge, short needle is inserted between the tendons. If a paresthesia is obtained, 3 to 5 ml of solution is injected; if none is obtained, a similar amount is injected in a fanlike manner between the two tendons.

Needle Puncture—Radial Block. To block the radial nerve at the wrist requires infiltration of its multiple peripheral branches that descend along the dorsal and radial aspect of the wrist. A field block is performed at the subcutaneous level in and around the anatomic "snuff box." The injection should be carried out superficial to the extensor pollicis longus tendon, which is easily identified by having the patient extend the thumb. This block may require from 5 to 6 ml of local anesthetic and is an infrequently used technique.

Potential Problems. As outlined, problems with the peripheral blocks primarily involve the potential for compression nerve injury and the suggestion of a slightly increased incidence of neuropathy following peripheral blockade. Theoretically, this occurs because of the tight fascial compartments in which these nerves run through the distal arm, forearm, and wrist. Likewise, blocking these distal nerves does not allow for tourniquet use, which is often the clinically limiting factor.

Figure 6–4 Wrist blocks—functional anatomy

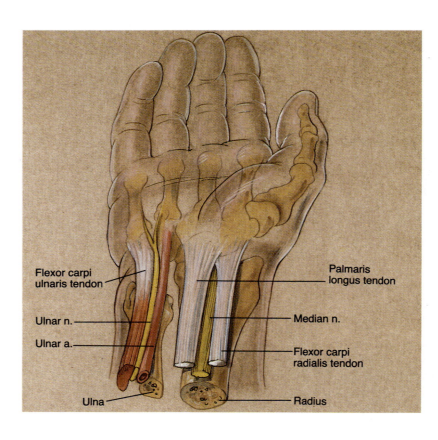

Flexor carpi ulnaris tendon

Ulnar n.

Ulnar a.

Ulna

Palmaris longus tendon

Median n.

Flexor carpi radialis tendon

Radius

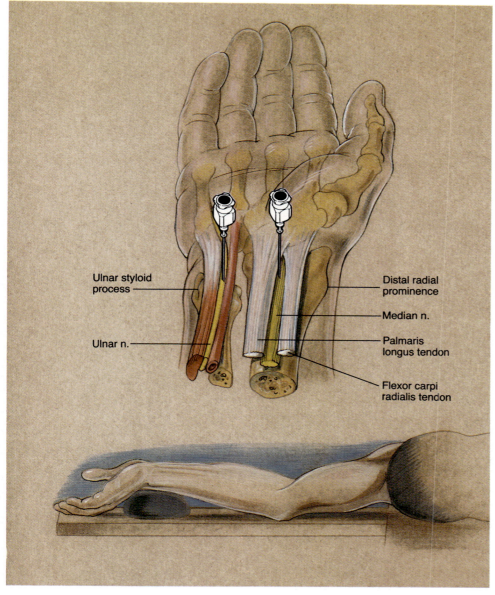

Figure 6—5 Wrist blocks—needle insertion and arm positioning

Ulnar styloid process

Ulnar n.

Distal radial prominence

Median n.

Palmaris longus tendon

Flexor carpi radialis tendon

Pearls

Suggestions for the successful use of these blocks involve avoiding them, when possible. Understanding the concepts outlined in axillary nerve blockade should make the necessity for the use of these blocks infrequent.

Digital Nerve Block

Perspective

Digital nerve block is a commonly employed block in emergency departments; however, it is an infrequently used block by anesthesiologists. It can be used for any surgery that requires a digital operation. However, its widest use is in repair of lacerations.

Patient Selection. Again the most common use for this block is in emergency department patients, although its use may be appropriate in an occasional elective surgical patient with a single digit surgical problem.

Pharmacologic Choice. As with any of the more peripheral upper extremity blocks, lower concentrations of any of the amide local anesthetics are appropriate for digital block, with the strong recommendation to avoid epinephrine-containing solutions.

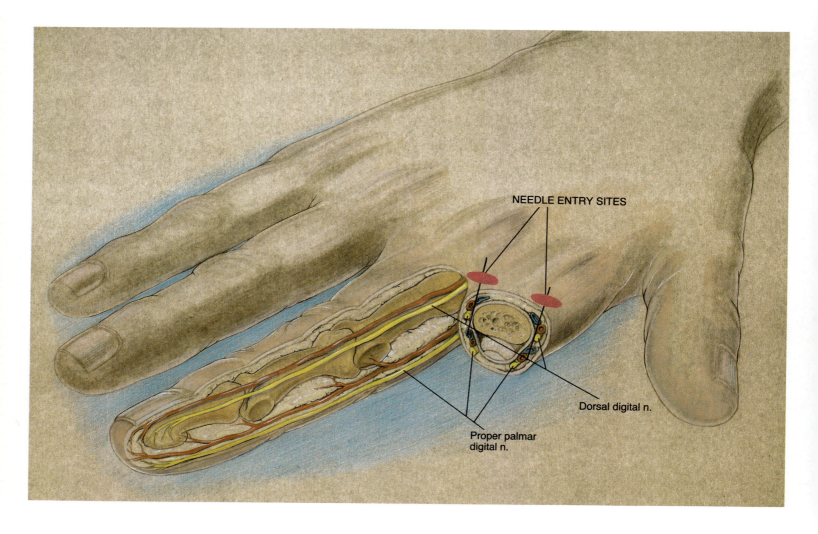

NEEDLE ENTRY SITES

Dorsal digital n.

Proper palmar
digital n.

Figure 6–6 Digital
block—anatomy and
needle insertion

Placement

Anatomy. As illustrated in Figure 6–6,
digital nerves can be conceptualized running
at the "corners" of the proximal phalanx.
The nerves run near arteries and veins and
are the distal continuation of both median
and ulnar nerves.

Position. Digital nerve block is most effectively carried out with the hand pronated.
The skin over the dorsum of the finger is less
tightly fixed to the underlying structures than
it is on the ventral surface of the digit.

Needle Puncture. Skin wheals are raised at
the dorsolateral borders of the proximal phalanx, and a blunt-beveled, small-gauge short
needle is inserted at the dorsal surface of the

lateral border of the phalanx. Infiltration of
both the dorsal and ventral branches of the
digital nerve is carried out bilaterally, and a
total of 1 to 2 ml at each site should be sufficient for blockade.

Potential Problems. It is emphasized once
again that epinephrine-containing solutions
should not be utilized for digital nerve block.

Pearls

These blocks should be used principally
for emergency department procedures, and
comprehensive anesthesia care requires at
least familiarity with the technique.

7

Intravenous Regional Block

Perspective

Intravenous regional anesthesia was introduced by Bier in 1908. As illustrated in Figure 7–1, the initial description required a surgical procedure to cannulate a vein and used both proximal and distal tourniquets to contain the local anesthetic in the venous system. After its introduction, the technique fell into disuse until the lower toxicity amino amides became available in the mid 1900s. This technique can be used for a variety of upper extremity operations, including both soft tissue and orthopedic procedures, primarily in the hand and forearm. The technique has also been used for foot procedures with a calf tourniquet.

Patient Selection. The technique is best suited for patients in whom there is no disruption of the venous system of the involved upper extremity, since the technique relies on an intact venous system. It can be used for distal orthopedic fractures and soft tissue operations. Intravenous regional block may not be appropriate for patients in whom movement of the upper extremity causes significant pain, since movement of the upper extremity is required to exsanguinate blood from the venous system adequately.

Pharmacologic Choice. The most commonly used agent for intravenous regional anesthesia is a dilute concentration of lidocaine; however, prilocaine has also been successfully used. Lidocaine is used in a 0.5% concentration, with approximately 50 ml used for an upper extremity intravenous regional block.

Placement

Anatomy. The only anatomic detail necessary for clinical use of the IV regional block is identification of a peripheral vein; one must be cannulated in the involved extremity.

Position. The patient should be resting supine upon the operating table with an IV already established in the nonsurgical arm. The involved arm should be extended on an arm board near available supplies, as illustrated in Figure 7–2.

Needle Puncture. Prior to placement of the intravenous line in the operative extremity, a tourniquet, either double or single, should be placed around the upper arm of the patient. An intravenous cannula is then inserted in the operative extremity, as distal as possible, most commonly in the dorsum of the hand (Fig. 7–3). There are two methods for exsanguination of the venous blood from the operative extremity. The traditional technique requires the wrapping of an Esmarch bandage from distal to proximal (Fig. 7–4). When the Esmarch bandage is not available or the patient is in too much pain to allow its placement, another method is to raise the arm for 3 to 4 minutes to allow gravity to exsanguinate the operative upper extremity (Fig. 7–5). After the blood has been exsanguinated from the upper extremity, the tourniquet is inflated. If a single tourniquet is in use, it is inflated; however, if a double tourniquet is in use, the upper tourniquet is inflated at this point. Recommendations for tourniquet inflation range from 50 mm Hg

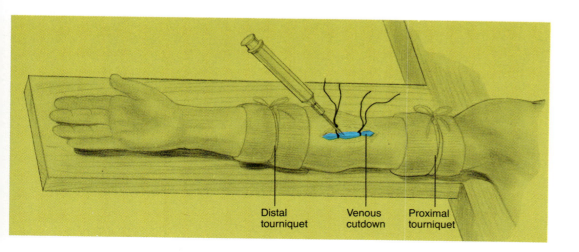

Figure 7–1 Early Bier block—surgical technique

Distal tourniquet   Venous cutdown   Proximal tourniquet

Figure 7–2 Intravenous regional block equipment

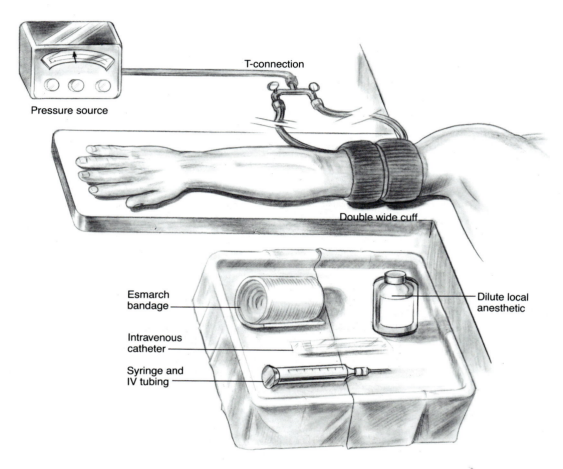

Pressure source

T-connection

Double wide cuff

Esmarch bandage

Intravenous catheter

Syringe and IV tubing

Dilute local anesthetic

Figure 7–3 Intravenous regional block—distal IV site

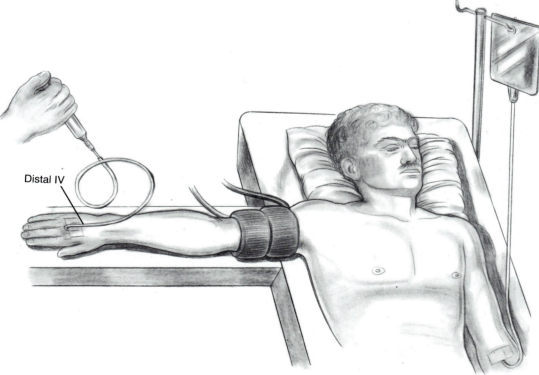

Distal IV

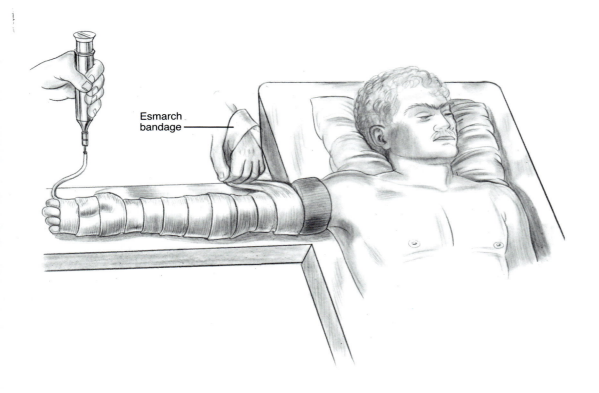

Figure 7—4 Intravenous regional block—venous exsanguination with Esmarch bandage

Esmarch
bandage

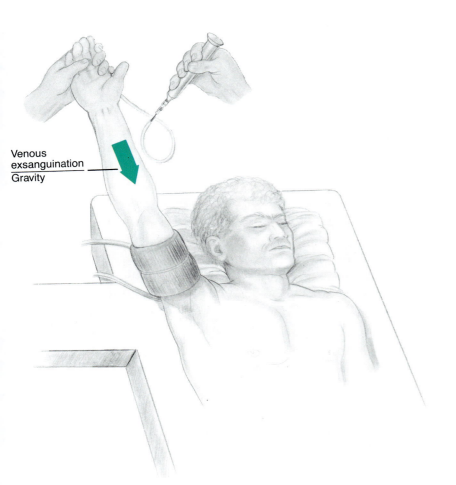

Figure 7—5 Intravenous regional block—venous exsanguination by gravity

Venous
exsanguination
Gravity

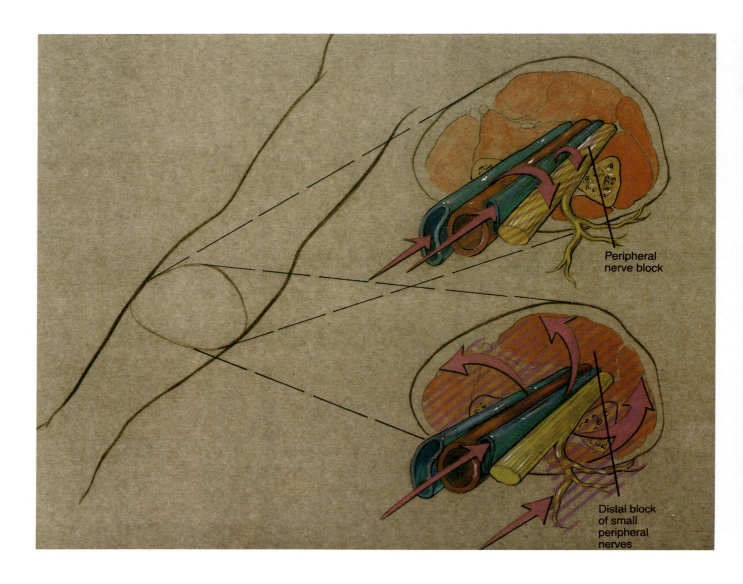

Peripheral
nerve block

Distal block
of small
peripheral
nerves

Figure 7–6 Intravenous regional block—potential mechanism(s) of action

above systolic blood pressure with a wide cuff, to a cuff pressure double the systolic blood pressure, to 300 mm Hg regardless of blood pressure. Until more information is available, I caution against using pressures greater than 300 mm Hg during upper extremity block.

If an Esmarch bandage has been used, the elastic bandage is then unwrapped, and in the average adult 50 ml of 0.5% lidocaine without a vasoconstrictor is injected. Onset of the block is usually within 5 minutes and the block is effective for procedures lasting as long as 90 to 120 minutes. This time limit is

due to tourniquet time constraints rather than to diminution of local anesthetic effect. The intravenous cannula is removed prior to preparation for operation. The block will persist as long as the cuff is inflated and disappears shortly following deflation.

Potential Problems. The principal disadvantage of intravenous regional anesthesia is that physicians unfamiliar with treating local anesthetic toxicity may use the technique when appropriate resuscitation measures are not available. Although some workers report successful use of intravenous regional anesthesia for lower extremity surgery, especially if a calf tourniquet is employed for foot surgery, its use is not widespread. During upper extremity use, a considerable number of patients will complain about tourniquet pressure even when a double tourniquet is used, and this is often the clinically limiting feature of this technique. Important for patient comfort is appropriate use of IV sedatives.

Pearls

Figure 7–6 illustrates the two complementary theories of how intravenous regional anesthesia produces blockade. The figure conceptualizes local anesthetic entering the venous system and producing blockade by blocking the peripheral nerves running with the venous structures. It also outlines a theory that may be complementary—that is, the local anesthetic leaves the veins and blocks small distal branches of peripheral nerves. It is likely that both of these theories are operative. If intravenous regional anesthesia is to be successfully used, all members of the operating team should understand the importance of tourniquet integrity, since the most significant problems with the technique involve unintentional deflation of the tourniquet.

8

Lower Extremity Anatomy

When lower extremity regional block is contrasted with upper extremity regional block, it is clear that anesthesiologists are more comfortable carrying out the former. In large part this is due to the ease and simplicity of blocking the lower extremities with centroneuraxis techniques. Additionally, in no anatomic site outside the centroneuraxis are the lower extremity plexuses as compactly packaged as are the nerves to the upper extremity in the brachial plexus. If one com-pares the path of lower extremity nerves over the pelvic brim, in a fashion similar to the routing of brachial plexus over the first rib, it is clear from Figures 8–1 and 8–2 that the four major nerves to the lower extremity exit from four widely differing sites. Thus, regional block of the lower extremity necessarily focuses on blockade of individual peripheral nerves, and my approach to anatomy will follow that concept.

In considering lower extremity innerva-

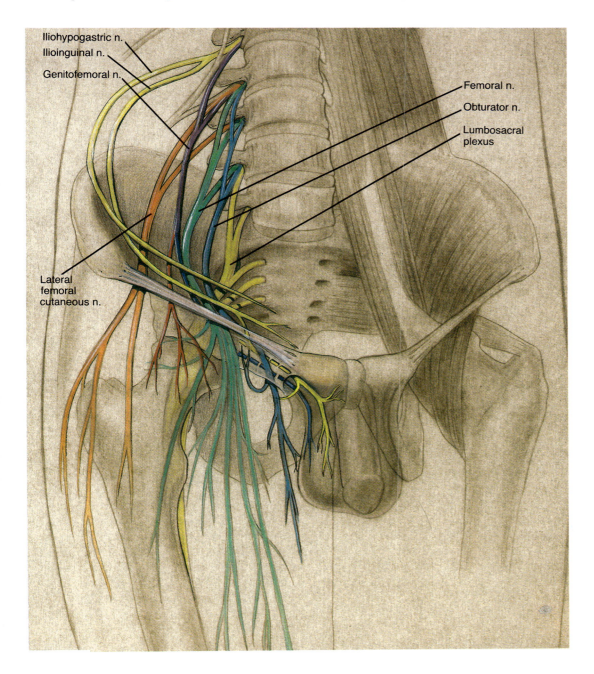

Figure 8–1 Lower extremity anatomy—major nerves—anterior oblique view

Iliohypogastric n.
Ilioinguinal n.
Genitofemoral n.
Femoral n.
Obturator n.
Lumbosacral plexus
Lateral femoral cutaneous n.

Figure 8–2 Lower extremity anatomy— major nerves—lateral view

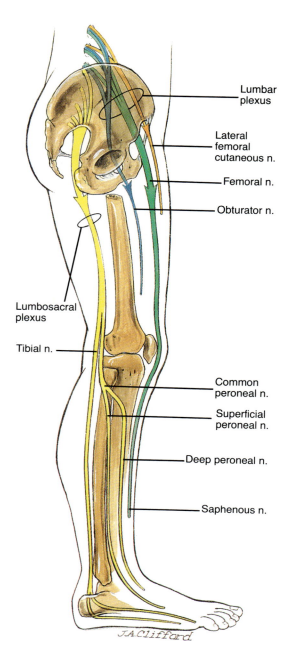

Lumbar plexus

Lateral femoral cutaneous n.

Femoral n.

Obturator n.

Lumbosacral plexus

Tibial n.

Common peroneal n.

Superficial peroneal n.

Deep peroneal n.

Saphenous n.

J.A.Clifford

tion, it is essential to understand that two major nerve plexuses innervate the lower extremity: the lumbar plexus and the lumbosacral plexus. The lumbar plexus is primarily involved in innervating the ventral aspect, whereas the lumbosacral plexus is primarily involved with innervating the dorsal aspect of the lower extremity (Fig. 8–2).

The lumbar plexus is formed from the ventral rami of the first three lumbar nerves and part of the fourth lumbar nerve. In approximately half of patients, a small branch from the 12th thoracic nerve joins the first lumbar nerve. The lumbar plexus forms from the ventral rami of these nerves anterior to the transverse processes of the lumbar vertebrae deeply within the psoas muscle (Fig. 8–3). The cephalic portion of the lumbar plexus—that is, the first lumbar nerve (and often a portion of the 12th thoracic nerve)— splits into superior and inferior branches. The superior branch re-divides into the iliohypogastric and ilioinguinal nerves, while the smaller inferior branch unites with a small superior branch of the second lumbar nerve to form the genitofemoral nerve (Fig. 8–1).

The *iliohypogastric nerve* penetrates the transversus abdominis muscle near the crest of the ilium and supplies motor fibers to the abdominal musculature. It ends in an anterior cutaneous branch to the skin of the suprapubic region and a lateral cutaneous branch in the hip region (Fig. 8–4).

The *ilioinguinal nerve* has a course slightly inferior to that of the iliohypogastric. It then traverses the inguinal canal and ends cutaneously in branches to the upper and medial parts of the thigh, and near the anterior scrotal nerves which supply the skin at the root of the penis and the anterior part of the scrotum in the male (Fig. 8–4). In women, the comparable anterior labial nerves supply the skin of the mons pubis and labia majora.

The *genitofemoral nerve* divides at a variable level into genital and femoral branches. The genital branch is small; it enters the inguinal canal at the deep inguinal ring and supplies the cremaster muscle, small branches to the skin and fascia of the scrotum, and adjacent parts of the thigh. The femoral branch is the more medial of the two branches and continues under the inguinal

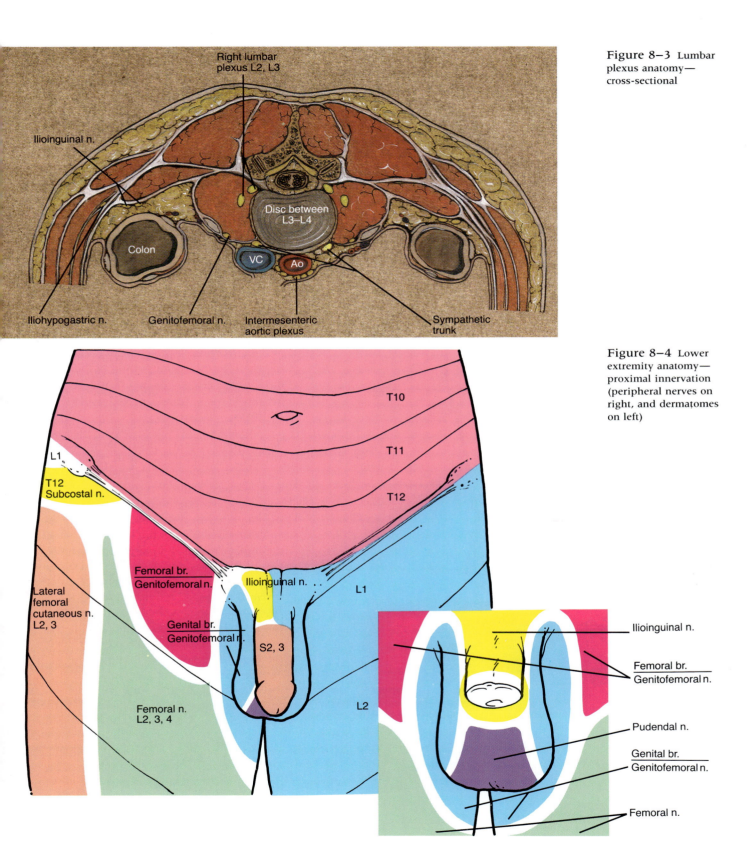

Figure 8–3 Lumbar plexus anatomy—cross-sectional

Right lumbar plexus L2, L3

Ilioinguinal n.

Disc between L3–L4

Colon

VC   Ao

Iliohypogastric n.   Genitofemoral n.   Intermesenteric aortic plexus   Sympathetic trunk

Figure 8–4 Lower extremity anatomy—proximal innervation (peripheral nerves on right, and dermatomes on left)

T10

T11

T12

L1

T12 Subcostal n.

Lateral femoral cutaneous n. L2, 3

Femoral br. Genitofemoral n.   Ilioinguinal n.

L1

Genital br. Genitofemoral n.

S2, 3

L2

Femoral n. L2, 3, 4

Ilioinguinal n.

Femoral br. Genitofemoral n.

Pudendal n.

Genital br. Genitofemoral n.

Femoral n.

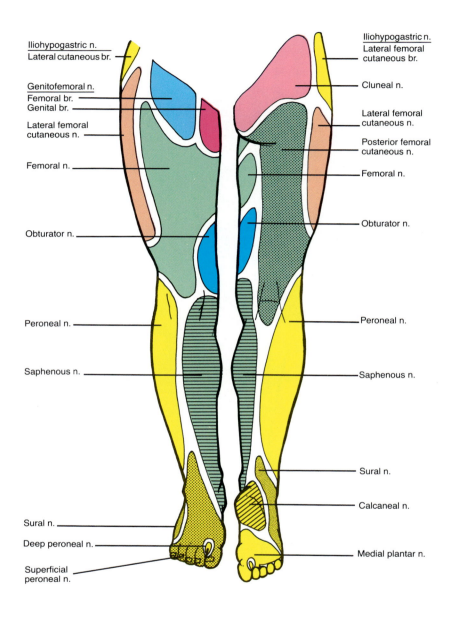

Iliohypogastric n.
Lateral cutaneous br.

Genitofemoral n.
Femoral br.
Genital br.

Lateral femoral
cutaneous n.

Femoral n.

Obturator n.

Peroneal n.

Saphenous n.

Sural n.

Deep peroneal n.

Superficial
peroneal n.

Iliohypogastric n.
Lateral femoral
cutaneous br.

Cluneal n.

Lateral femoral
cutaneous n.

Posterior femoral
cutaneous n.

Femoral n.

Obturator n.

Peroneal n.

Saphenous n.

Sural n.

Calcaneal n.

Medial plantar n.

Figure 8–5 Lower
extremity anatomy—
proximal and distal
innervation

ligament on the anterior surface of the external iliac artery. Below the inguinal ligament, it pierces the femoral sheath and passes via the saphenous opening to supply the skin over the femoral triangle lateral to that supplied by the ilioinguinal nerve (Fig. 8–4). These three nerves are clinically important during regional block for inguinal herniorrhaphy, or other groin procedures carried out under regional block.

Caudal to these three nerves are three major nerves of the lumbar plexus that exit from the pelvis anteriorly and innervate the lower extremity. These are lateral femoral cutaneous, femoral, and obturator nerves (see Figs. 8–1 and 8–2).

The *lateral femoral cutaneous nerve* passes under the lateral end of the inguinal ligament. It may be superficial or deep to the sartorius muscle, and it descends at first deep to the fascia lata. It provides cutaneous innervation to the lateral portion of the buttock distal to the greater trochanter and to the proximal two thirds of the lateral aspect of the thigh.

The *obturator nerve* descends along the medial posterior aspect of the psoas muscle and descends through the pelvis to the obturator canal into the thigh. This nerve supplies the adductor group of muscles, the hip and knee joints, and the skin on the medial aspect of the thigh proximal to the knee.

The *femoral nerve* is the largest branch of the lumbar plexus. It emerges through the fibers of the psoas muscle at the muscle's lower lateral border and descends in the groove between the psoas and iliacus muscles. It passes under the inguinal ligament within this groove. Slightly prior to, or upon, entering the femoral triangle of the upper thigh, the femoral nerve breaks into numerous branches supplying the muscles and skin of the anterior thigh, knee, and hip joints.

The lumbosacral plexus is formed by the ventral rami of the lumbar fourth and fifth and sacral first, second, and third nerves. Occasionally, a portion of the fourth sacral nerve contributes to the sacral plexus. The nerve from the plexus of primary interest to anesthesiologists during lower extremity blockade is the sciatic nerve. The posterior femoral cutaneous nerve is sometimes listed as an additional branch important to anes-

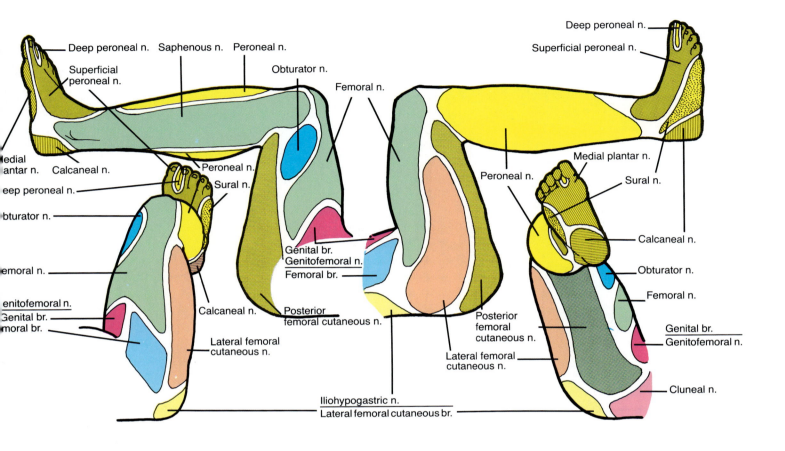

Deep peroneal n.   Saphenous n.   Peroneal n.

Superficial peroneal n.

Obturator n.

Femoral n.

Deep peroneal n.

Superficial peroneal n.

Medial plantar n.

Peroneal n.

Sural n.

Medial plantar n.   Calcaneal n.

Deep peroneal n.

Obturator n.

Femoral n.

Genitofemoral n.
Genital br.
Femoral br.

Peroneal n.

Sural n.

Genital br.
Genitofemoral n.
Femoral br.

Calcaneal n.

Posterior femoral cutaneous n.

Genital br.
Genitofemoral n.

Posterior femoral cutaneous n.

Lateral femoral cutaneous n.

Calcaneal n.

Obturator n.

Femoral n.

Lateral femoral cutaneous n.

Genital br.
Genitofemoral n.

Iliohypogastric n.
Lateral femoral cutaneous br.

Cluneal n.

thesiologists. In reality the sciatic nerve is the combination of two major nerve trunks: the first is the tibial nerve, derived from the anterior branches of the ventral rami of the fourth and fifth lumbar and first, second, and third sacral nerves, whereas the second major portion of the sciatic nerve is the common peroneal nerve, derived from the dorsal branches of the ventral rami of the same five nerves. These two major nerve trunks pass as the sciatic through the upper leg to the popliteal fossa, where they divide into their terminal branches, tibial and common peroneal.

Figure 8–5 illustrates the cutaneous innervation of the peripheral nerves of the lower extremity. I have chosen to illustrate this with the patient's lower extremity in both the anatomic and the lithotomy positions. These should provide a unique and clinically useful perspective. Likewise, Figures 8–6 and 8–7 illustrate the dermatomal innervation of the lower extremities in a similar manner. Figure 8–8 illustrates the osteotome pattern of lower extremity innervation and will be most useful to the anesthesiologists who are providing anesthesia for orthopedic procedures. Figure 8–9 helps provide an understanding of cross-sectional anatomy pertinent to regional block of the lower extremity.

Figure 8–6 Lower extremity anatomy in lithotomy position—proximal and distal peripheral nerves

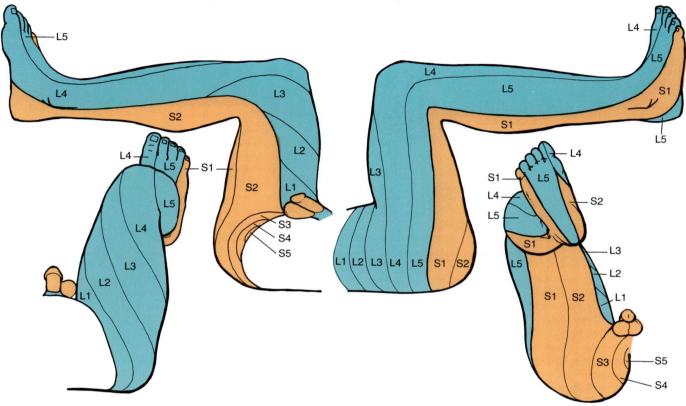

Figure 8–7 Lower extremity anatomy in lithotomy position— dermatomes

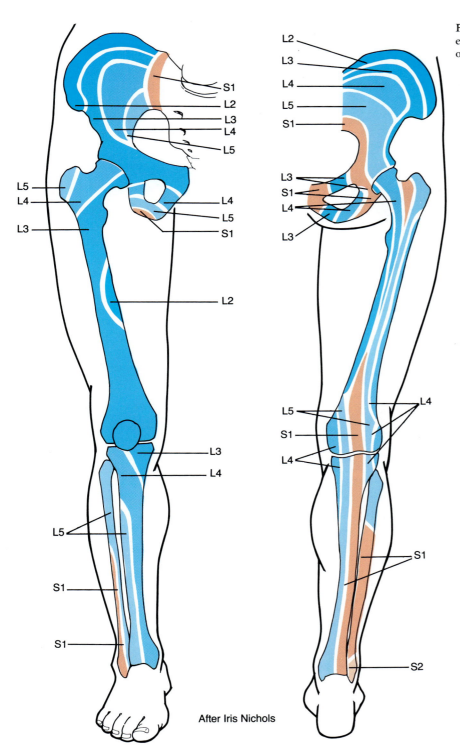

Figure 8—8 Lower extremity anatomy—osteotomes

After Iris Nichols

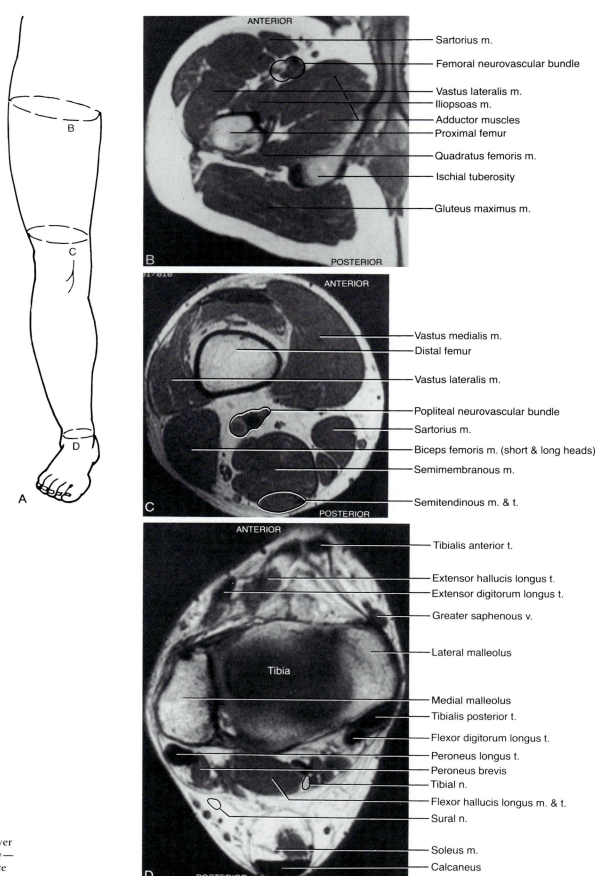

Figure 8–9 Lower extremity anatomy— magnetic resonance cross-sectional images

Sartorius m.

Femoral neurovascular bundle

Vastus lateralis m.
Iliopsoas m.
Adductor muscles
Proximal femur

Quadratus femoris m.

Ischial tuberosity

Gluteus maximus m.

Vastus medialis m.
Distal femur

Vastus lateralis m.

Popliteal neurovascular bundle
Sartorius m.
Biceps femoris m. (short & long heads)
Semimembranous m.

Semitendinous m. & t.

Tibialis anterior t.

Extensor hallucis longus t.
Extensor digitorum longus t.

Greater saphenous v.

Lateral malleolus

Tibia

Medial malleolus
Tibialis posterior t.
Flexor digitorum longus t.
Peroneus longus t.
Peroneus brevis
Tibial n.
Flexor hallucis longus m. & t.
Sural n.

Soleus m.
Calcaneus

ANTERIOR
POSTERIOR
ANTERIOR
POSTERIOR
ANTERIOR
POSTERIOR

A
B
C
D

9

Lumbar Plexus Block

Inguinal Perivascular Block (3-in-1 Block)

Perspective

The inguinal perivascular block is based on the concept of injecting local anesthetic near the femoral nerve in an amount sufficient to track proximally along fascial planes to anesthetize the lumbar plexus. The three principal nerves of the lumbar plexus pass from the pelvis anteriorly: the lateral femoral cutaneous, the femoral, and the obturator nerve. As illustrated in Figure 9–1, the theory behind this block presumes that the local anesthetic will track in the fascial plane between the iliacus and psoas muscles to reach the region of the lumbar plexus roots.

Patient Selection. As outlined, lower extremity blockade is often most effectively and efficiently performed with centroneuraxis blocks. Nevertheless, in some patients avoidance of bilateral blockade and/or sympathectomy may make an alternative approach necessary.

Pharmacologic Choice. Local anesthetics should be selected by deciding whether primarily sensory or sensory and motor blockade is needed. Any of the amino amides can be used. It has been suggested that the volume of local anesthetic needed for adequate lumbar plexus block from this approach can be estimated by dividing the patient's height, in inches, by three. That number is the volume of local anesthetic in milliliters that theoretically will provide lumbar plexus blockade.

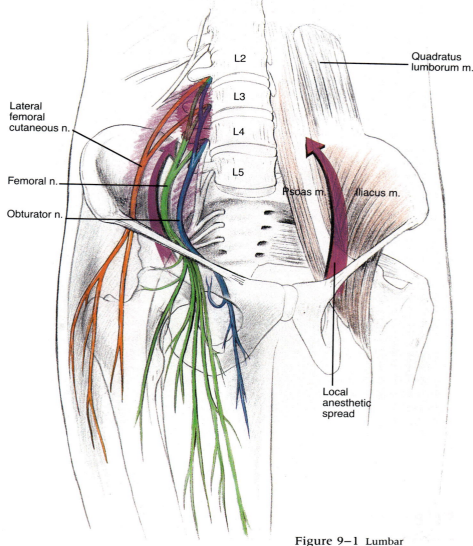

Figure 9–1 Lumbar plexus anatomy—proposed mechanism of proximal local anesthetic spread

Placement

Anatomy. The concept behind this block is that the only anatomy one needs to visualize is the extension of sheathlike fascial planes that surround the femoral nerve.

Position. The patient should be placed supine on the operating table with the anesthesiologist standing at the patient's side in position to palpate the ipsilateral femoral artery.

Needle Puncture. A short-beveled, 22-gauge, 5-cm needle is inserted immediately lateral to the femoral artery, caudal to the inguinal ligament in the lower extremity to be blocked. It is advanced with cephalic angula-tion until a femoral paresthesia is obtained. At this point the needle is firmly fixed, and, while the distal femoral sheath is digitally compressed, the entire volume of local anesthetic is injected.

Potential Problems. My clinical experience suggests that the principal problem with this technique is a lack of predictability. Additionally, whenever a large volume of local anesthetic is injected through a fixed, "immobile" needle, risk of systemic toxicity is increased. If the technique is used, incremental injection of local anesthetic, accompanied by frequent aspiration for blood, should be carried out.

Pearls

My suggestion is to use this block when lower extremity analgesia is the goal, rather than choosing it when anesthesia is needed for operation. I do not believe one needs to master this technique to provide comprehensive regional anesthesia care.

Psoas Compartment Block

Perspective

In concept, the psoas compartment block produces blockade of all lumbar and some sacral nerves, thus providing anesthesia of the anterior thigh. If anesthesia to the lower leg or posterior thigh is needed for the procedure, sciatic block must be added.

Patient Selection. Again, in the usual clinical situation a centroneuraxis block is more effective, and more time-efficient in producing lower extremity block. However, as emphasized for the inguinal perivascular block, there may be patients in whom avoidance of bilateral lower extremity blockade and/or the sympathectomy accompanying centroneuraxis block is desirable.

Pharmacologic Choice. When selecting a local anesthetic, consideration must be given to

degree of motor and sensory block required, with realization that a total of approximately 30 ml of local anesthetic is suggested for use with the block. Again, any of the amino amides may be chosen.

Placement

Anatomy. As Figure 9-2 identifies, the nerves of the lumbar plexus can be anesthetized by depositing solution in the psoas compartment, which is immediately posterior to the psoas muscle and anterior to the transverse process of the fifth lumbar vertebra.

Position. The patient should be placed in a lateral decubitus position with thighs flexed upon the trunk, similar to that for centroneuraxis block, with the operative extremity uppermost. The anesthesiologist should be positioned in a fashion similar to that necessary for lumbar subarachnoid puncture.

Needle Puncture. With patient in position, a line is drawn between the iliac crests—i.e., Tuffier's line. The vertebral spine palpable on this line in the midline is most often the fourth lumbar spine. The midline is marked on this line, and a second line is made 5 cm lateral to the midline parasagittally on the side to be anesthetized. On this second line, a mark is made 3 cm caudal to a line joining the iliac crests (Tuffier's line), and this identi-

Figure 9–2 Psoas compartment—functional anatomy

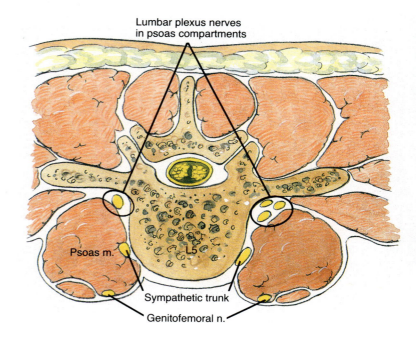

Lumbar plexus nerves in psoas compartments

Psoas m.

L5

Sympathetic trunk

Genitofemoral n.

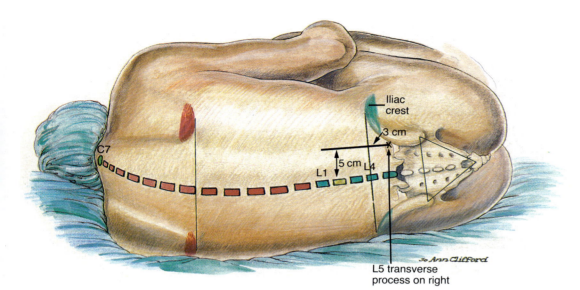

Figure 9–3 Psoas compartment block— surface anatomy

fies the needle entry site (Fig. 9-3). At this point, a 20-gauge, 15-cm needle is inserted, as illustrated in Figure 9-4, to the depth of the transverse process of the fifth lumbar vertebra (position 1). Once the transverse process is located, the needle is partially withdrawn and redirected cephalad until it slides past the transverse process. The original description suggests attaching a 20-ml air-containing syringe to the needle and slowly advancing it until loss of resistance is achieved. The needle tip is then within the psoas compartment (position 2). The loss of resistance typically occurs at a depth of 12 ± 2 cm.

If the needle placement is in question, the needle can be farther advanced until resistance is once again encountered (within psoas muscle mass), and then the needle is withdrawn until loss of resistance is appreciated a second time. At this point the needle is again in the psoas compartment. Once the psoas compartment has been identified, 20 ml of air is injected to dilate the space, followed by 30 ml of local anesthetic. The patient is kept in the lateral position for 5 minutes following completion of local anesthetic injection.

Potential Problems. As with any single fascial compartment injection of local anesthetic, local anesthetic toxicity risk is increased. Also, insertion of the needle near the centroneuraxis makes possible epidural or subarachnoid injection. Pain from lumbar paravertebral muscle spasm can be troublesome postoperatively.

Pearls

This block is technically easy to perform, although considerable sedation is necessary to make patients comfortable. Similar to the inguinal perivascular block, this approach seems more suited for providing analgesia than anesthesia. In addition, as outlined for the inguinal perivascular block, comprehensive regional anesthesia is possible without mastering this technique.

Figure 9–4 Psoas compartment block— needle insertion— cross sectional and parasagittal anatomy

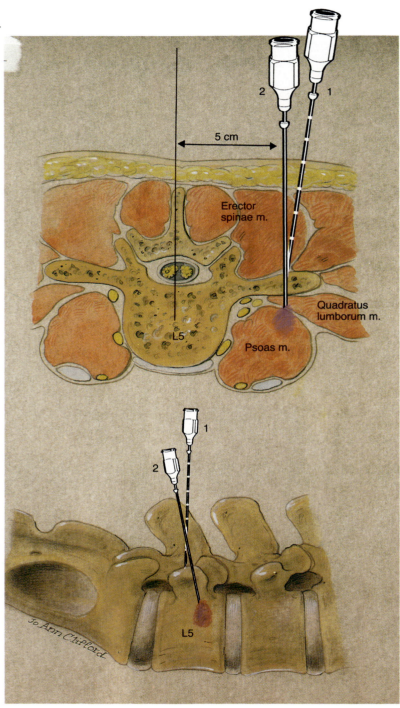

Sciatic Block

Perspective

The sciatic nerve is one of the largest nerve trunks in the body, yet few surgical procedures can be performed with sciatic block alone. It is most often combined with femoral, lateral femoral cutaneous, and/or obturator nerve blocks to produce surgical anesthesia of the lower leg. The block is also effective for analgesia of the lower leg and may provide pain relief from ankle fractures or tibial fractures prior to operative intervention.

Patient Selection. This block may be indicated for patients needing analgesia prior to transport for definitive orthopedic surgical repair of lower leg or ankle fractures. There also may be patients in whom it is desirable to avoid the sympathectomy accompanying centroneuraxis block, and in these patients sciatic block combined with femoral nerve block often allows ankle and foot procedures to be carried out. One group of patients in whom this is often useful are those undergoing distal amputations of the lower extremity, whose vascular compromise is based on diabetes or peripheral vascular disease.

Pharmacologic Choice. Sciatic nerve block requires from 20 to 25 ml of local anesthetic solution. When this volume is added to that required for other lower extremity peripheral blocks, the total may reach the upper end of acceptable local anesthetic dose range. Conversely, uptake of local anesthetic from these lower extremity sites is not as rapid as with epidural or intercostal blockade; thus, larger mass of local anesthetic may be appropriate in this region. If motor blockade is desired with this block, 1.5% mepivacaine or lidocaine may be necessary, whereas 0.5% bupivacaine will be effective.

Placement

Anatomy. The sciatic nerve is formed from L-4 through S-3 roots. These roots of the sacral plexus form on the anterior surface of the lateral sacrum and are assembled into the sciatic nerve on the anterior surface of the piriform muscle. The sciatic nerve results from the fusion of two major nerve trunks: The "medial" sciatic nerve is functionally the tibial nerve, which forms from the ventral

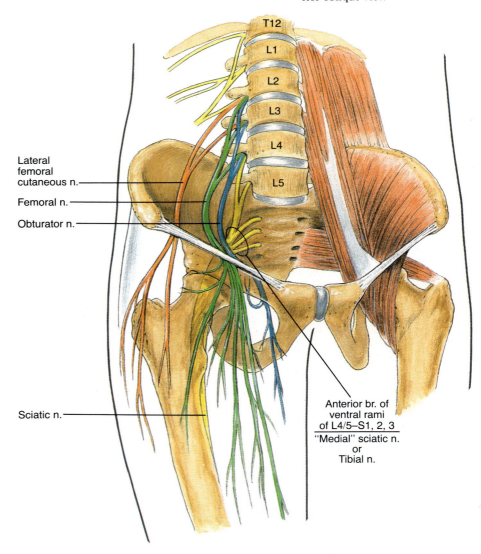

Figure 10–1 Sciatic nerve anatomy—anterior oblique view

T12
L1
L2
L3
L4
L5

Lateral femoral cutaneous n.
Femoral n.
Obturator n.
Sciatic n.

Anterior br. of ventral rami of L4/5–S1, 2, 3
"Medial" sciatic n.
or
Tibial n.

Figure 10–2 Sciatic nerve anatomy—posterior view

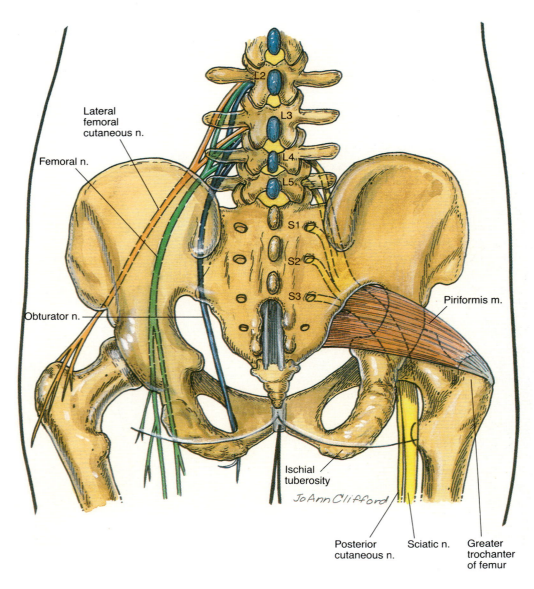

Lateral femoral cutaneous n.

Femoral n.

Obturator n.

L2

L3

L4

L5

S1

S2

S3

Piriformis m.

Ischial tuberosity

JoAnn Clifford

Posterior cutaneous n.

Sciatic n.

Greater trochanter of femur

branches of the ventral rami of L-4/5 and S-1–3. The posterior branches of the ventral rami of these same nerves form the "lateral" sciatic nerve, which is functionally the peroneal nerve. As the sciatic nerve exits from the pelvis, it is anterior to the piriformis muscle and is joined by a nerve, the posterior cutaneous nerve of the thigh. At the inferior border of the piriformis, the sciatic and posterior cutaneous nerves of the thigh lie posterior to the obturator internus, the gemelli, and the quadratus femoris. At this point, these nerves are anterior to the gluteus maximus. Here, the nerve is approximately equidistant from the ischial tuberosity and the

greater trochanter (Figs. 10–1, 10–2, and 10–3). The nerve continues on a downward course through the thigh to lie along the posterior medial aspect of the femur. At the cephalad portion of the popliteal fossa, the sciatic nerve usually divides to form the tibial and common peroneal nerves. Occasionally this division occurs much higher, and sometimes the tibial and peroneal nerves are separate through their entire course. In the popliteal fossa, the tibial nerve continues its downward course into the lower leg, while the common peroneal nerve travels laterally along the medial aspect of the short head of the biceps femoris muscle.

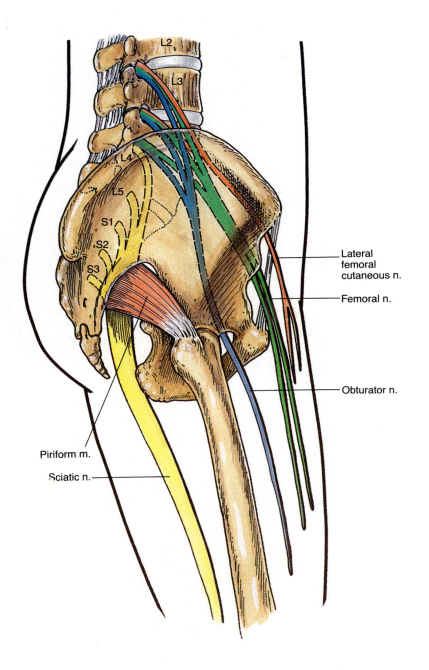

Figure 10–3 Sciatic nerve anatomy—lateral view

Lateral femoral cutaneous n.

Femoral n.

Obturator n.

Piriform m.

Sciatic n.

Classic Approach—Sciatic Block

Position. The patient is positioned laterally, with the side to be blocked nondependent. The flexed, nondependent leg supports the patient by placement of the heel of the nondependent leg opposed to the knee of the dependent leg (Fig. 10–4). The anesthesiologist is positioned to allow insertion of the needle, as shown in Figure 10–4.

Needle Puncture. A line is drawn from the posterior superior iliac spine to the midpoint of the greater trochanter. Perpendicular to the midpoint of this line, another line is extended caudomedially for 5 cm. The needle is inserted through this point. As a cross-check for proper placement, an additional line may be drawn from the sacral hiatus to the previously marked point on the greater trochanter. The intersection of this line with the 5-cm perpendicular line should coincide with the needle insertion site (Fig. 10–5).

Through this site, a 22-gauge, 10- to 12-cm needle is inserted, as illustrated in Figure 10–4. The needle should be directed through the entry site toward an imaginary point where the femoral vessels course under the inguinal ligament. The needle is inserted until a paresthesia is elicited, or until bone is contacted. If bone is encountered prior to eliciting a paresthesia, the needle is redirected along the line joining the sacral hiatus and the greater trochanter until paresthesia is elicited. During this needle redirection, the needle should not be inserted more than 2 cm past the depth at which bone was originally contacted, or the needle tip will be placed anterior to the site of the sciatic nerve. Once a paresthesia is elicited, 20 to 25 ml of local anesthetic is injected.

Potential Problems. In patients in whom the block is being used for injury to the lower extremity, the classic position is sometimes difficult to use. This block can also be long

Figure 10–4 Sciatic nerve block—classic technique and positioning

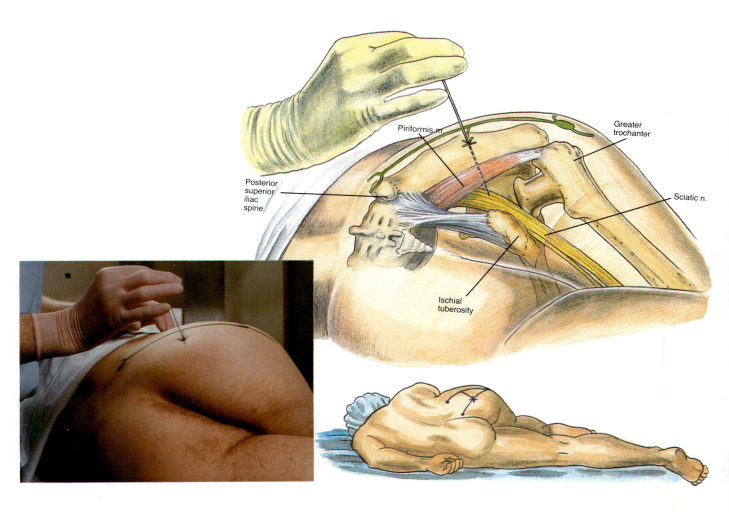

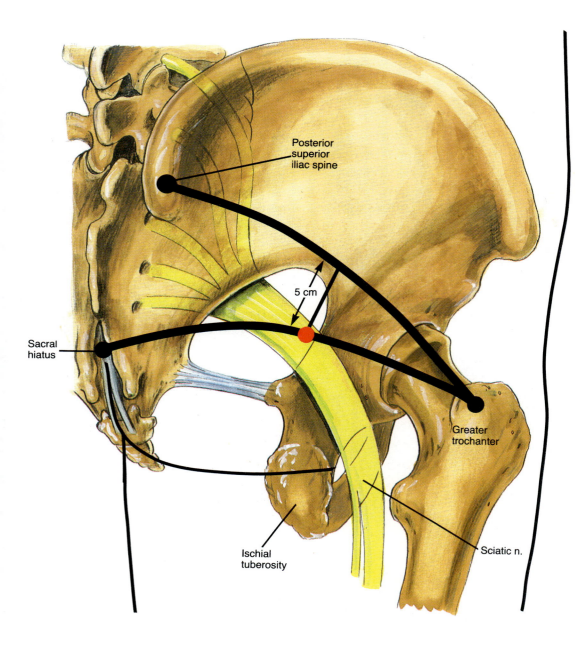

Figure 10–5 Sciatic nerve block—technique of surface markings

Posterior superior iliac spine

5 cm

Sacral hiatus

Greater trochanter

Sciatic n.

Ischial tuberosity

lived, and patients should be warned of this preoperatively to prevent undue concern postoperatively. It is unsubstantiated, but some consider that dysesthesias may be more common after this block than after other peripheral blocks.

Pearls

The keys to making this block work are adequate positioning of the patient and a systematic redirection of the needle until a paresthesia is obtained.

Anterior Approach—Sciatic Block

Position. The anterior block of the sciatic nerve can be carried out in the supine patient whose leg is in the neutral position. The anesthesiologist should be at the patient's side, similar to positioning during femoral nerve block.

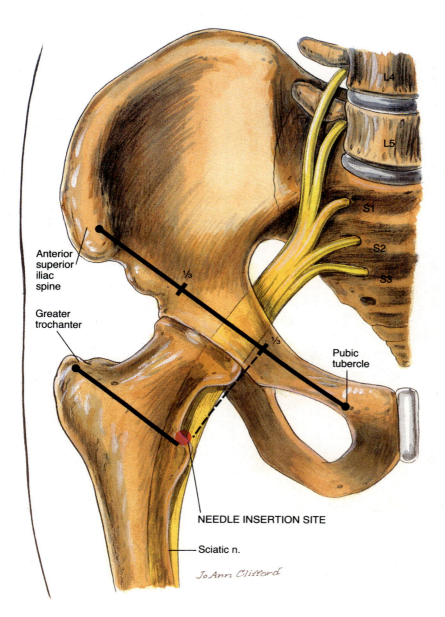

Needle Puncture. In the supine patient, a line should be drawn from the anterior superior iliac spine to the pubic tubercle. Another line should be drawn parallel to this line from the midpoint of the greater trochanter inferomedially, as illustrated in Figure 10–6. The first line is trisected, and a perpendicular line is drawn caudolaterally from the juncture of the medial and middle thirds, as shown in Figure 10–6. At the point where the perpendicular line crosses the more caudal line, a 22-gauge, 12-cm needle is inserted so that it contacts the femur at its medial border. Once the needle has contacted the femur, it is redirected slightly medially to slide off the medial surface of the femur. At approximately 5 cm past the depth required to contact the femur, a paresthesia should be sought to insure successful blockade (Fig. 10–7). Once a paresthesia is obtained, 20 to 25 ml of local anesthetic is injected.

Potential Problems. The same problems that exist for the classic approach need to be considered with this anterior approach.

Pearls

This block has the advantage of a simple concept; however, my ability to produce anesthesia with the anterior approach is considerably less than my ability with the classic approach to the sciatic nerve. Perhaps, with additional experience, this difference would not be as apparent. This block may be useful in supine patients who are in significant discomfort and cannot be positioned for the classic approach.

Anterior
superior
iliac
spine

Greater
trochanter

Pubic
tubercle

NEEDLE INSERTION SITE

Sciatic n.

JoAnn Clifford

Figure 10–6 Sciatic nerve block—anterior technique

ANTERIOR

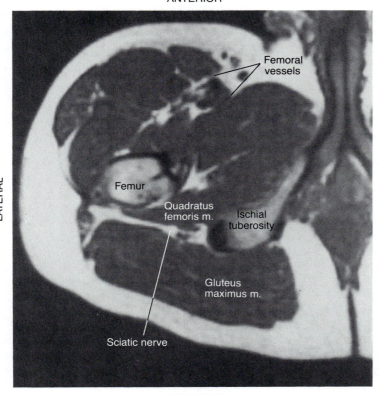

LATERAL

Femoral
vessels

Femur

Quadratus
femoris m.

Ischial
tuberosity

Gluteus
maximus m.

Sciatic nerve

POSTERIOR

Figure 10–7 Magnetic resonance image (cross-sectional) at level of anterior sciatic nerve

11

Femoral Block

Perspective

This block is useful for surgical procedures carried out on the anterior thigh, both superficial and deep. It is most frequently combined with other lower extremity peripheral blocks to provide anesthesia for operation on the lower leg and foot. As an analgesic technique, it is used for femur fracture analgesia.

Patient Selection. Since the patient is in the supine position when this block is carried out, virtually any patient undergoing a surgical procedure of the lower extremity is a candidate for this block. Paresthesias are not necessary to carry out this block; thus, even anesthetized patients are candidates for femoral block.

Pharmacologic Choice. As with all lower extremity blocks, a decision must be made about the extent of sensory and motor blockade desired. If motor blockade is necessary, higher concentrations of local anesthetic will be necessary. As with concerns for sciatic local anesthetic use, the desire for motor blockade must be considered in light of the volume of local anesthetic necessary if femoral, sciatic, lateral femoral cutaneous, and obturator blocks are combined. Approximately 20 ml of local anesthetic should be adequate to produce femoral blockade.

Placement

Anatomy. The femoral nerve travels through the pelvis in the groove between the psoas and the iliacus muscles, as illustrated in Figure 11–1. It emerges beneath the inguinal ligament, posterolateral to the femoral vessels, as illustrated in Figure 11–2. It fre-

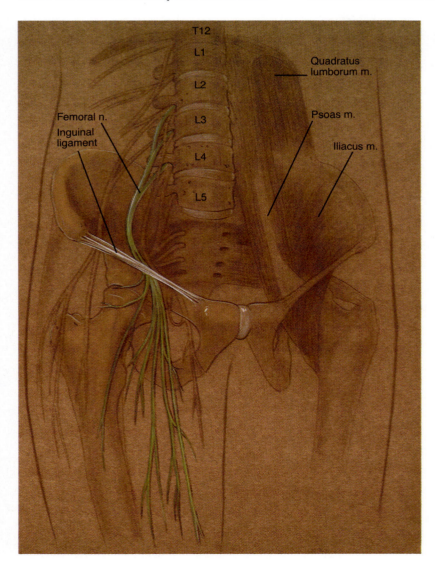

Figure 11–1 Femoral nerve anatomy— anterior oblique view

T12
L1
L2
L3
L4
L5

Quadratus lumborum m.

Psoas m.

Iliacus m.

Femoral n.
Inguinal ligament

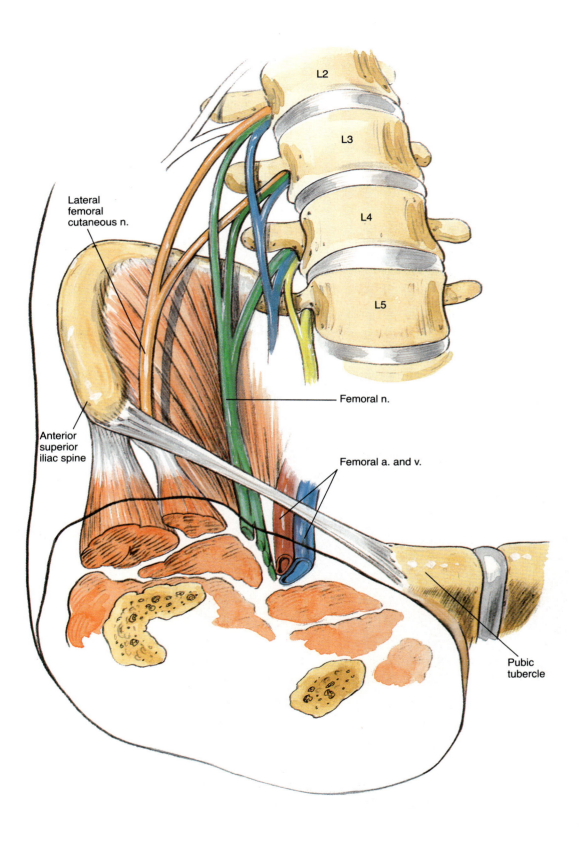

Figure 11–2 Femoral nerve anatomy—at inguinal ligament

Lateral femoral cutaneous n.

Anterior superior iliac spine

L2

L3

L4

L5

Femoral n.

Femoral a. and v.

Pubic tubercle

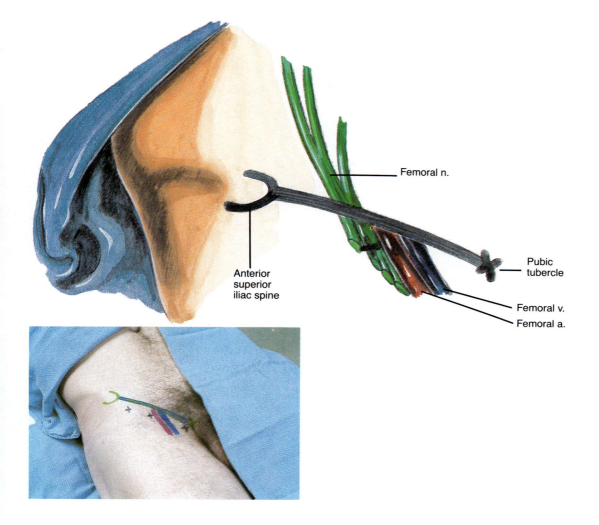

Figure 11–3 Femoral nerve block—technique

Femoral n.

Anterior
superior
iliac spine

Pubic
tubercle

Femoral v.
Femoral a.

quently divides into its branches at or above the level of the inguinal ligament.

Position. The patient is in a supine position, and the anesthesiologist should stand at the patient's side to allow easy palpation of the femoral artery.

Needle Puncture. A line is drawn connecting the anterior superior iliac spine and the pubic tubercle, as illustrated in Figure 11–3. The femoral artery is palpated on this line, and a 22-gauge, 4-cm needle is inserted, as illustrated in Figure 11–4. The initial insertion should abut the femoral artery in a perpendicular fashion, as shown in Figure 11–5 (position 1), and in a fanlike manner a "wall" of local anesthetic is developed by redirecting the needle in progressive steps to position 2. Approximately 20 ml of local anesthetic is injected incrementally in this fash-

ion. It may also be useful to displace the needle entry site laterally 1 cm, direct the needle tip to lie immediately posterior to the femoral artery, and inject an additional 2 to 5 ml of drug. This allows blockade of those fibers that may be in a more posterior relationship to the femoral artery. Elicitation of paresthesias is variable with this block; however, if one does occur, the medial to lateral injection should still be carried out, since the nerve often divides into branches cephalic to the inguinal ligament.

Potential Problems. Unilateral lower extremity blockade is often indicated for patients with peripheral vascular disease; thus, a number of patients with prosthetic femoral arteries may be suitable candidates for this block. If lower extremity peripheral regional blockade has been chosen in a patient who

Figure 11—4 Femoral nerve block—technique

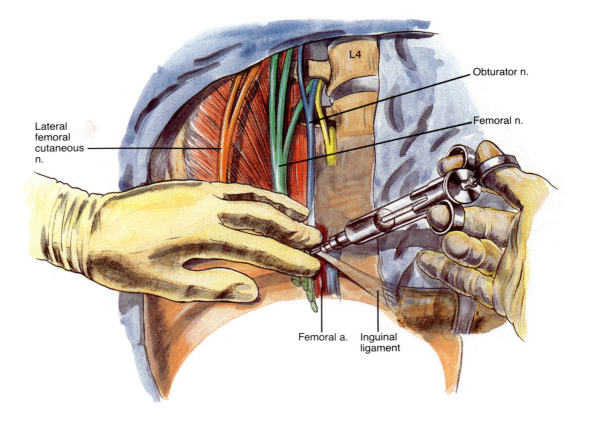

Lateral femoral cutaneous n.

L4

Obturator n.

Femoral n.

Femoral a. Inguinal ligament

has recently undergone placement of a prosthetic femoral artery, efforts should be made to avoid the newly placed prosthesis.

Pearls

Since this block is actually a field block, enough "soak time" must be allowed to produce satisfactory anesthesia. When combining sciatic and femoral block, it is often helpful to place the femoral block prior to the sciatic block, thus allowing extra soak time.

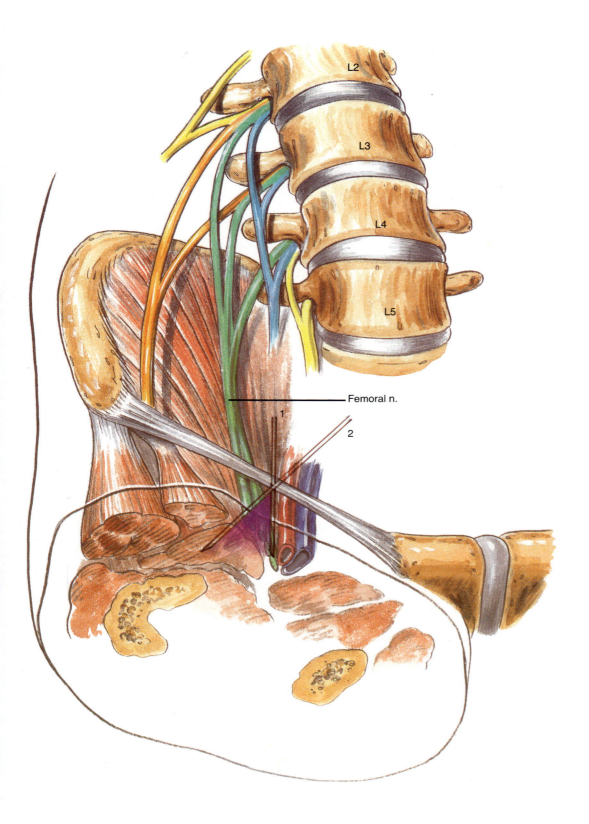

L2

L3

L4

L5

Femoral n.

1

2

Figure 11–5 Femoral nerve block—technique of local anesthetic injection

Lateral Femoral Cutaneous Block

Perspective

When this block is combined with other lower extremity blocks, it allows lower leg procedures to be carried out with fewer complaints of tourniquet pain. It also allows superficial procedures upon the lateral thigh, including skin graft harvesting. In your pain practice, it allows the diagnosis of myalgia paresthetica, which is a neuralgia involving the lateral femoral cutaneous nerve.

Patient Selection. Like femoral nerve block, this block is carried out with the patient in the supine position. Thus, almost any patient is a candidate for a lateral femoral cutaneous block.

Pharmacologic Choice. The same concerns about local anesthetic choice that were outlined in sciatic and femoral block apply to the lateral femoral cutaneous blockade. If multiple nerves to the lower extremity are to be blocked, be aware of the mass of drug utilized. Conversely, this nerve does not have

motor components; thus, a lower concentration of 10 to 15 ml of local anesthetic is effective.

Placement

Anatomy. As shown in Figure 12–1, the lateral femoral cutaneous nerve emerges along the lateral border of the psoas muscle immediately caudal to the ilioinguinal nerve. It courses deep to the iliac fascia and anterior to the iliacus muscle to emerge from the fascia immediately inferior and medial to the anterior superior iliac spine, as shown in Figure 12–2. After passing beneath the inguinal ligament, it crosses or passes through the origin of the sartorius muscle and travels beneath the fascia lata, dividing into anterior and posterior branches at variable distances below the inguinal ligament. The anterior branch supplies skin over the anterolateral thigh, whereas the posterior branch supplies

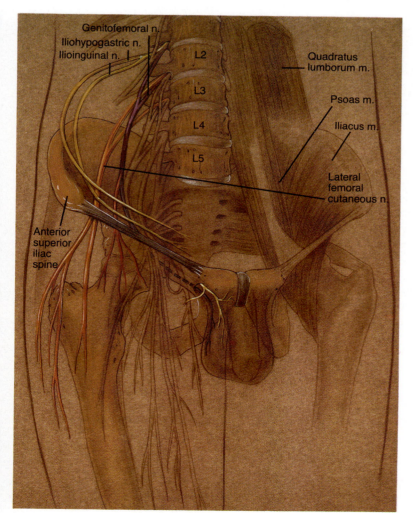

Figure 12–1 Lateral femoral cutaneous nerve—anatomy

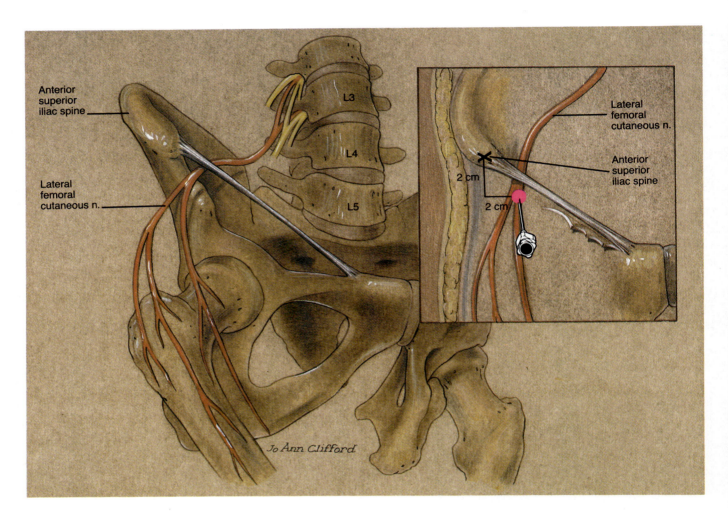

Figure 12−2 Lateral femoral cutaneous nerve block—technique

the skin over the lateral thigh from the greater trochanter to mid thigh.

Position. The patient is in a supine position with the anesthesiologist at the patient's side, similar to that for femoral nerve block.

Needle Puncture. The anterior superior iliac spine is marked in the supine patient, and a 22-gauge, 4-cm needle is inserted at a site 2 cm medial and 2 cm caudal to the mark (Fig. 12−2). As shown in Figure 12−3, the needle is advanced until a pop is felt as the needle passes through the fascia lata. Local anesthetic is then injected in a fanlike manner above and below the fascia lata, from medial to lateral, as illustrated in Figure 12−3.

Potential Problems. The superficial nature

of this block allows one to avoid most problems associated with regional blockade.

Pearls

An adequate volume of local anesthetic should be used for this block—that is, 10 to 15 ml. Since this is a sensory nerve, low concentrations of local anesthetics are useful—that is, 0.5% to 0.75% mepivacaine and lidocaine or 0.25% bupivacaine. By keeping the concentration lower for this portion of a "three- or four-nerve" lower extremity block, adequate volumes and concentrations of local anesthetic can be maintained for the sciatic and femoral nerves.

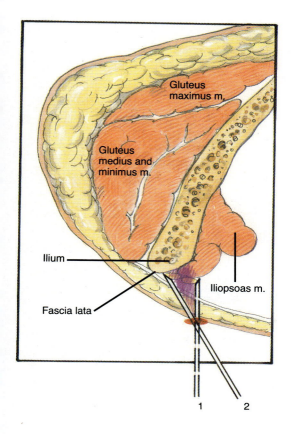

Figure 12–3 Lateral femoral cutaneous nerve—cross-sectional technique of local anesthetic injection

13

Obturator Block

Perspective

This block is most often combined with the sciatic, femoral, and lateral femoral cutaneous blocks to allow surgical procedures upon lower extremities. If an operation upon the knee using these blocks is planned, the obturator block is often essential. Another use for this block is in patients who have hip pain. It can be used diagnostically to help identify the cause of pain, since blockade of the obturator nerve may provide considerable pain relief if the obturator's articular branch to the hip is involved in pain transmission. Additionally the block may be useful in evaluation of lower extremity spasticity.

Patient Selection. As with femoral and lateral femoral cutaneous nerve blocks, elicitation of paresthesias is not essential for obturator blockade. Any patient able to lie supine is a candidate.

Pharmacologic Choice. Motor blockade is most often not necessary for patients receiving obturator nerve block; thus, lower concentrations of local anesthetics are appropriate for obturator block—i.e., 0.75% to 1.0% lidocaine, 0.75% to 1.0% mepivacaine, and 0.25% bupivacaine.

Placement

Anatomy. The obturator nerve emerges from the medial border of the psoas muscle at the pelvic brim and travels along the lateral aspect of the pelvis anterior to the obturator internus muscle and posterior to the iliac vessels and ureter. It enters the obturator canal cephalic and anterior to the obturator vessels, which are branches from the internal iliac vessels. In the obturator canal, the obturator nerve divides into anterior and posterior branches (Fig. 13–1.) The anterior

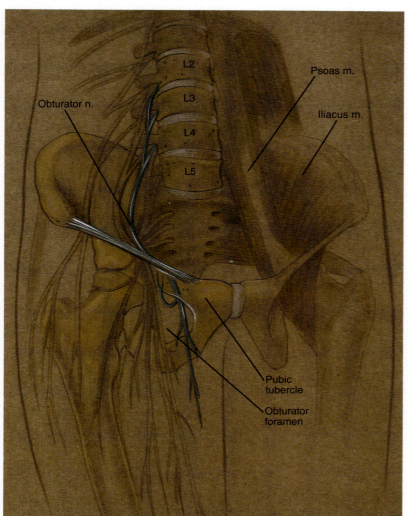

Figure 13–1 Obturator nerve—functional anatomy

Obturator n.

L2

L3

L4

L5

Psoas m.

Iliacus m.

Pubic tubercle

Obturator foramen

branch supplies anterior adductor muscles, as well as an articular branch to the hip joint and a cutaneous area on the medial aspect of the thigh. The posterior branch innervates the deep adductor muscles and sends an articular branch to the knee joint. In 10% of patients, an accessory obturator nerve may be found.

Position. The patient should be supine, with the legs positioned in a slightly abducted position. The genitalia should be protected from antiseptic solutions.

Needle Puncture. The pubic tubercle should be located and an **X** marked 1.5 cm caudal and 1.5 cm lateral to the tubercle (Fig. 13–2). At this point the needle is inserted, and at a depth of approximately 1.5 to 4 cm

the horizontal ramus of the pubis will be contacted. The needle is then withdrawn and redirected laterally in a horizontal plane and inserted 2 to 3 cm deeper than the depth of the initial contact of bone. The needle tip now lies within the obturator canal (Fig. 13–3). With the needle in this position, 10 to 15 ml of local anesthetic solution is injected while advancing and withdrawing the needle slightly to assure developing a "wall" of local anesthetic in the canal.

Potential Problems. The obturator canal is a vascular location; thus, the potential exists for intravascular injection or hematoma formation, although these are more theoretical than clinical concerns.

Figure 13–2 Obturator nerve anatomy—oblique view

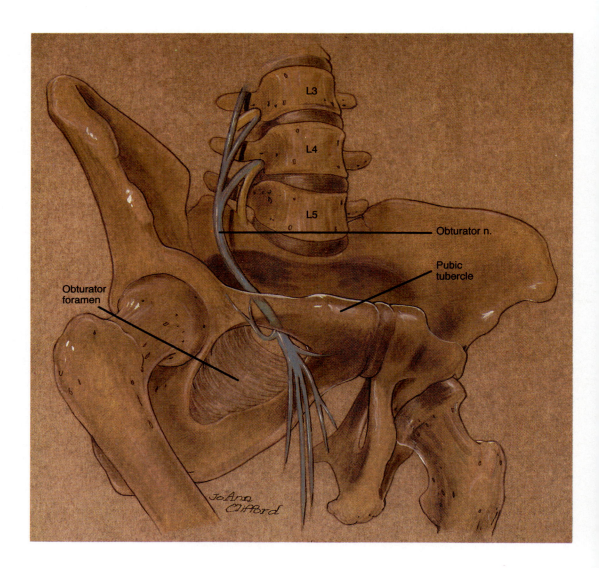

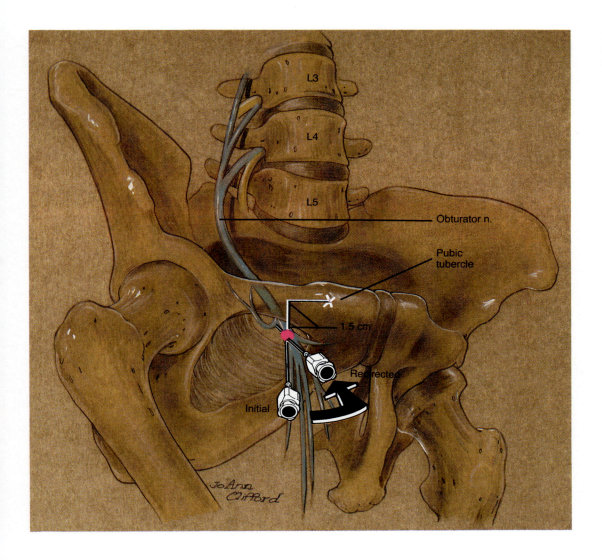

Figure 13–3 Obturator nerve block—technique

Pearls

This block, even in trained hands, has a variable success rate. My experience suggests that one must rely on volume for this block, rather than on "rifle-like" accuracy of needle position. Fortunately, the necessity to use obturator block with the other lower extremity peripheral nerve blocks is not an absolute.

14

Popliteal Block

Perspective

The nerves blocked in the popliteal fossa—that is, tibial and peroneal nerves—are extensions of the sciatic nerve. The principal use of this block is for foot and ankle surgery.

Patient Selection. To utilize this block, the patient must be able to assume the prone position. Although elicitation of a paresthesia is desirable, it is not essential, though block effectiveness decreases without paresthesias.

Pharmacologic Choice. The principal use of these blocks is to provide sensory analgesia; thus, lower concentrations of local anesthetic are practical in contrast to situations in which motor blockade is essential. One per cent lidocaine, 1% mepivacaine, and 0.25% to 0.5% bupivacaine are effective.

Placement

Anatomy. As illustrated in Figure 14–1, the popliteal fossa is defined cephalically by the semimembranous and semitendinous muscles medially and the biceps femoris muscle laterally. Its caudal extent is defined by the gastrocnemius muscles both medially and laterally. If this quadrilateral is bisected, as shown in Figure 14–1, the area of interest to the anesthesiologist is the cephalolateral quadrant. Here both tibial and common peroneal nerve blockade is possible. The tibial nerve is the larger of the two nerves; it separates from the common peroneal nerve at the upper limit of the popliteal fossa, and sometimes higher. The tibial nerve continues the straight course of the sciatic nerve and runs lengthwise through the popliteal fossa direct-

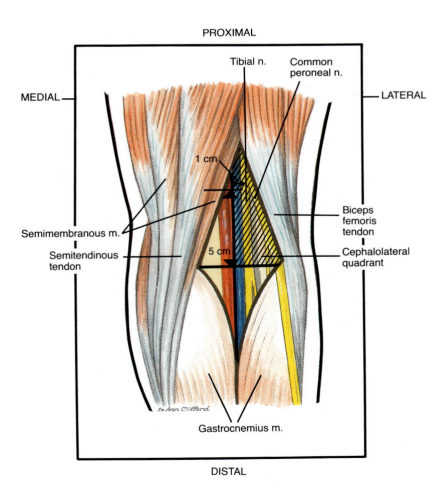

Figure 14–1 Popliteal fossa surface anatomy and technique

ly under the popliteal fascia. Inferiorly it passes between the heads of the gastrocnemius muscles. The common peroneal nerve follows the tendon of the biceps femoris muscle along the cephalic lateral margin of the popliteal fossa, as illustrated in Figure 14–2. After the common peroneal nerve leaves the popliteal fossa, it travels around the head of the fibula and divides into the superficial peroneal and deep peroneal nerves.

Position. The patient is in a prone position and the anesthesiologist stands at the patient's side to allow palpation of the borders of the popliteal fossa.

Needle Puncture. With the patient in the prone position, the patient is asked to flex the leg at the knee, which allows more accurate identification of the popliteal fossa. Once

the popliteal fossa is defined, it is divided into equal medial and lateral triangles, as shown in Figure 14–1. An **X** is placed 5 cm superior to the skin crease of the popliteal fossa and 1 cm lateral to the mid line of the triangles, as shown in Figure 14–1. Through this site, a 22-gauge, 4- to 6-cm needle is advanced at an angle of 45° to 60° to the skin, while the needle is directed anterosuperiorly (Fig. 14–3). A paresthesia is sought, and, if obtained, 30 to 40 ml of local anesthetic is injected.

Potential Problems. Although vascular structures also occupy the popliteal fossa, intravascular injection should be an infrequent occurrence if usual precautions are carried out. Hematoma formation is possible.

Figure 14–2 Popliteal fossa—neural anatomy

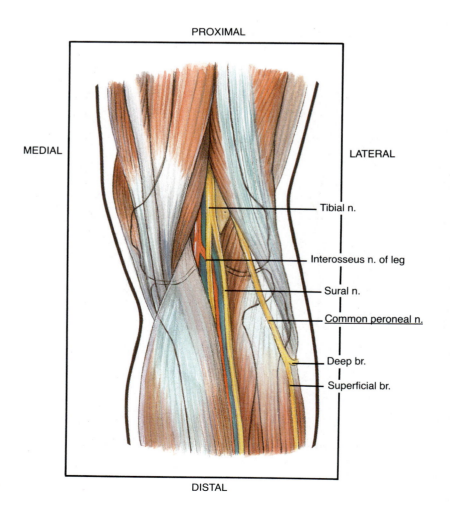

PROXIMAL

MEDIAL

LATERAL

Tibial n.

Interosseus n. of leg

Sural n.

Common peroneal n.

Deep br.

Superficial br.

DISTAL

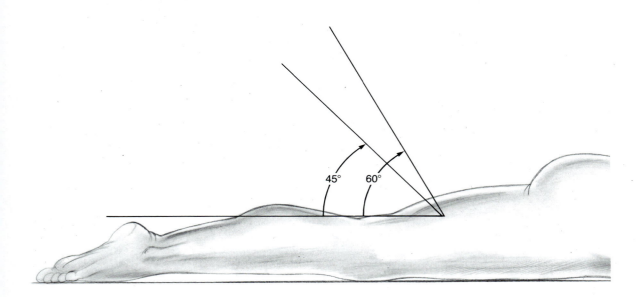

Pearls

There is an interesting dichotomy of interest in popliteal nerve blockade. Very favorable reports emanate from the centers that utilize the block. Conversely, centers with considerable experience in regional anesthesia often seem disinterested in advancing this block. Whether this dichotomy is simply clinical bias or based on clinical efficacy remains to be established. As with many other lower extremity peripheral nerve blocks, volume seems to be the key in making this block useful.

Figure 14–3 Popliteal fossa technique

15

Ankle Block

Perspective

This block is often used for surgical procedures carried out on the foot, especially for those not requiring high tourniquet pressure.

Patient Selection. The ankle block is principally an infiltration block, not requiring elicitation of paresthesia. Thus, patient cooperation is not mandatory for successful use of the block. Although the block is most efficient for the anesthesiologist if the patient can assume the prone as well as supine positions, this is not absolutely essential for performance of the block.

Pharmacologic Choice. Since motor blockade is not often needed for procedures carried out during ankle blockade, lower concentrations of local anesthetics may be utilized. One per cent lidocaine, 1% mepivacaine, or 0.25% to 0.5% bupivacaine is a practical choice. Many workers suggest that epinephrine should not be used during ankle block, especially if injection is circumferential.

Placement

Anatomy

The peripheral nerves requiring blockade during ankle block are all derived from the sciatic nerve, with the exception of a terminal branch of the femoral nerve, the saphenous. The saphenous nerve is the only branch of the femoral below the knee; it courses superficially anterior to the medial malleolus, providing cutaneous innervation to an area of the medial ankle and foot. The remaining nerves requiring blockade at the ankle are terminal branches of the sciatic—that is, common peroneal and tibial nerves. The tibial nerves divide into posterior tibial and sural nerves, which provide cutaneous innervation as outlined in Figure 15–1. The common peroneal nerve divides into its terminal branches in the proximal portion of the lower leg by dividing into the superficial and deep peroneal nerves. Their cutaneous innervation is also illustrated in Figure 15–1. Figure 15–2 identifies where these nerves are located in a cross-sectional view at the level of ankle block.

Needle Puncture

It is often helpful to have the patient in the prone position initially, so that blockade of the posterior tibial and sural nerves is facilitated. Once these two nerves have been blocked, the patient assumes the supine position so that blockade of the saphenous and peroneal nerves can be carried out. The block can be performed with the patient in the supine position if the foot is placed on a padded support.

Posterior Tibial Nerve. With the patient in the prone position, the ankle to be blocked is supported upon a pillow. A 22-gauge, 4-cm needle is directed anteriorly at the cephalic border of the medial malleolus, just medial to the Achilles tendon, as outlined in Figure 15–2. The needle is inserted near the posterior tibial artery, and, if a paresthesia is obtained, 3 to 5 ml of local anesthetic is injected. If no paresthesia is obtained, the needle is allowed to contact the medial malleolus, and 5 to 7 ml of local anesthetic is deposited near the posterior tibial artery.

Sural Nerve. The sural nerve is blocked with the patient positioned as for posterior tibial nerve block. As illustrated in Figure 15–2, blockade of the sural nerve is carried out by inserting a 22-gauge, 4-cm needle anterolaterally immediately lateral to the Achilles tendon at the cephalic border of the lateral malleolus. If no paresthesia is obtained, the needle is allowed to contact the lateral malleolus, and 5 to 7 ml of local anesthetic is injected as the needle is withdrawn.

Deep Peroneal, Superficial Peroneal, and Saphenous Nerves. After the patient assumes the supine position, the anterior tibial artery pulsation is located at the superior level of the malleoli. A 22-gauge, 4-cm needle is advanced posteriorly and immediately lateral to this point (Fig. 15–2). An alternative is to insert the needle between the tendons of the anterior tibial and extensor hallucis longus muscles. Approximately 5 ml of local anesthetic is injected in this area. From this midline skin wheal, a 22-gauge, 8-cm needle is advanced subcutaneously laterally and medially to the malleoli, injecting 3 to 5 ml of local anesthetic in each direction. These lateral and medial approaches block the superficial peroneal and saphenous nerves, respectively.

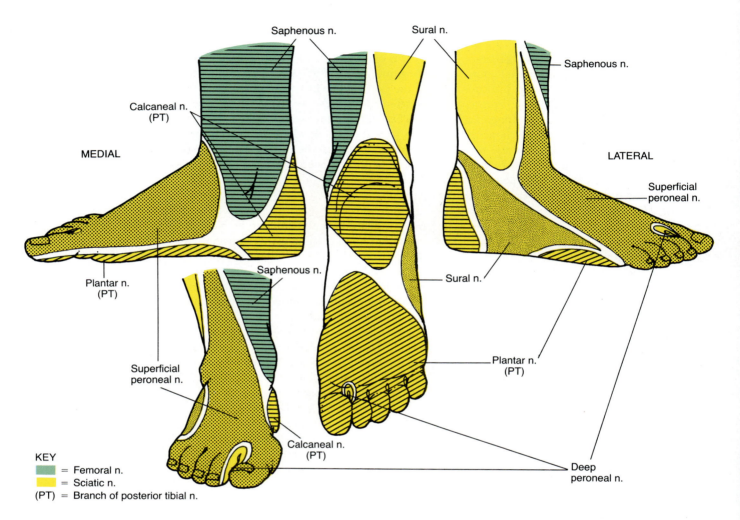

KEY
■ = Femoral n.
■ = Sciatic n.
(PT) = Branch of posterior tibial n.

Figure 15–1 Ankle block—peripheral innervation

Potential Problems

The ankle block can be painful if the patient is not adequately sedated, although this should be an infrequent problem because an alert patient is not essential for the block.

Pearls

As alluded to, patients should be adequately sedated during this block, since it is primarily a "volume" block. The block should not be chosen if high tourniquet pressures are required to carry out the surgical procedure. Again, epinephrine-containing solutions should be avoided in circumferential injections of the ankle. Following outpatient foot surgery, patients often can walk with assistance even after ankle block has been used. This is sometimes an advantage, since the stay of these patients in the outpatient surgery center generally is not unnecessarily prolonged, and they experience effective postoperative analgesia.

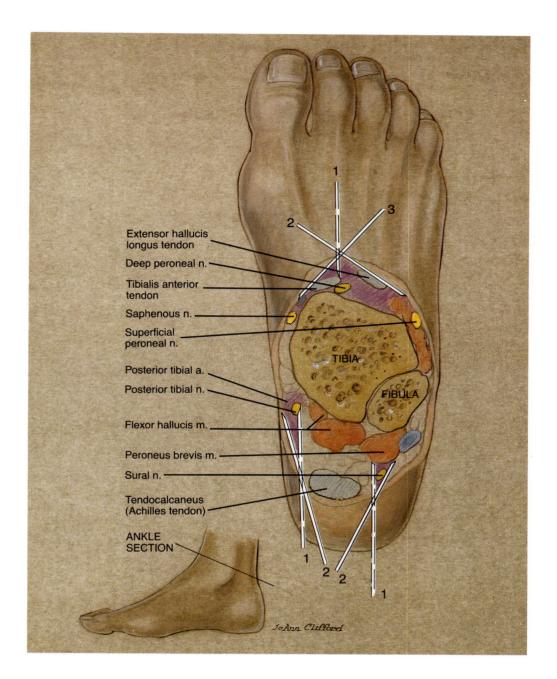

Extensor hallucis
longus tendon

Deep peroneal n.

Tibialis anterior
tendon

Saphenous n.

Superficial
peroneal n.

Posterior tibial a.

Posterior tibial n.

Flexor hallucis m.

Peroneus brevis m.

Sural n.

Tendocalcaneus
(Achilles tendon)

ANKLE
SECTION

TIBIA

FIBULA

JoAnn Clifford

Figure 15–2 Ankle block—cross-sectional anatomy and technique

16

Head and Neck Block Anatomy

Regional anesthesia for head and neck surgery declined rapidly after general anesthesia and tracheal intubation became available and accepted. Despite the decline in using regional anesthesia for head and neck surgery, in few other areas in the body can such small doses of local anesthetic provide such effective regional block. Likewise, one of the reasons head and neck blockade fell into disuse is that in no other body region can such small doses of local anesthetic produce systemic toxicity so easily. There are still circumstances in which head and neck blockade is useful. Many of these involve the diagnosis or treatment of pain syndromes. Also, many plastic surgical procedures upon superficial structures can be managed easily with effective blockade of nerves of the head and neck. One aspect of head and neck blockade that should not be considered optional for anesthesiologists is the develop-

ment of expertise in airway anatomy and innervation. In some circumstances in an anesthetic practice, proper airway management, including airway blockade, can be lifesaving.

Sensory innervation of the face is from the trigeminal nerve. Three branches of the trigeminal—ophthalmic, maxillary, and mandibular—provide innervation, as illustrated in Figure 16–1. The cutaneous innervation of the posterior head and neck is from the cervical nerves. The dorsal ramus of the second cervical nerve ends in the greater occipital nerve, which provides cutaneous innervation to the larger portion of the posterior scalp (Fig. 16–1). The greater occipital nerve is a continuation of the medial branch of the dorsal ramus of the second cervical nerve and ascends from the cervical vertebrae to the muscles of the neck in company with the occipital artery. The greater occipital nerve becomes subcutaneous in its course with the

Figure 16–1 Head and neck anatomy—innervation

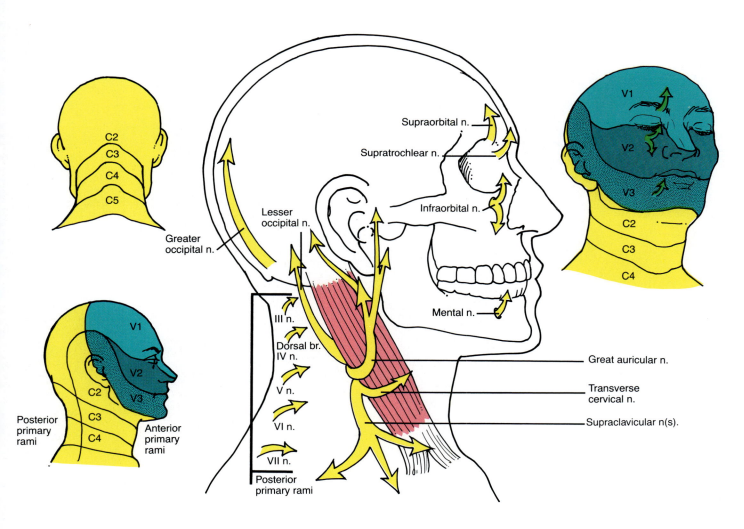

occipital artery immediately lateral to the inion, slightly inferior to the superior nuchal line (Fig. 16–2). The ventral rami of cervical nerves 2, 3, and 4 provide the majority of cutaneous innervation to the anterior and lateral portions of the neck, with cervical nerve 2 providing innervation to the scalp through both lesser occipital and posterior auricular nerves (see Fig. 16–1). The superficial cervical plexus is formed as cervical nerves 2, 3, and 4 leave the vertebral transverse processes and follow a course in which they become subcutaneous at the midpoint of the posterior border of the sternocleidomastoid muscle (Fig. 16–2). At this point, the superficial cervical plexus can be easily blocked by infiltration.

The trigeminal nerve is a mixed motor and sensory nerve, although the majority of it involves sensory innervation. The only motor fibers are the branches that supply the muscles of mastication, via the mandibular nerve. The trigeminal nerve is organized in the cranium within the trigeminal ganglion (gasserian or semilunar ganglion). From this ganglion, the ophthalmic nerve exits from the cranium via the superior orbital fissure; the maxillary nerve exits via the foramen rotundum; and the mandibular nerve via the foramen ovale (Fig. 16–3). The maxillary and mandibular nerves follow a course after leaving these foramina that places them in the immediate proximity of the lateral pterygoid plate. The pterygoid plate is an important landmark for effective maxillary or mandibular blockade (Fig. 16–4). The terminal branches of the trigeminal nerve end in the supraorbital, infraorbital, and mental nerves. These exit through bony foramina that fall on a perpendicular line through the pupil, as illustrated in Figure 16–5.

Figure 16–2 Head and neck anatomy—peripheral nerves

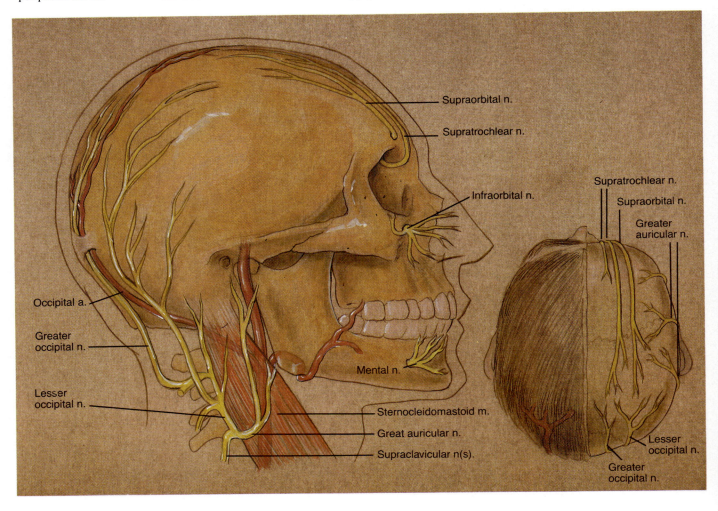

Supraorbital n.

Supratrochlear n.

Infraorbital n.

Supratrochlear n.

Supraorbital n.

Greater auricular n.

Occipital a.

Greater occipital n.

Mental n.

Lesser occipital n.

Sternocleidomastoid m.

Great auricular n.

Supraclavicular n(s).

Lesser occipital n.

Greater occipital n.

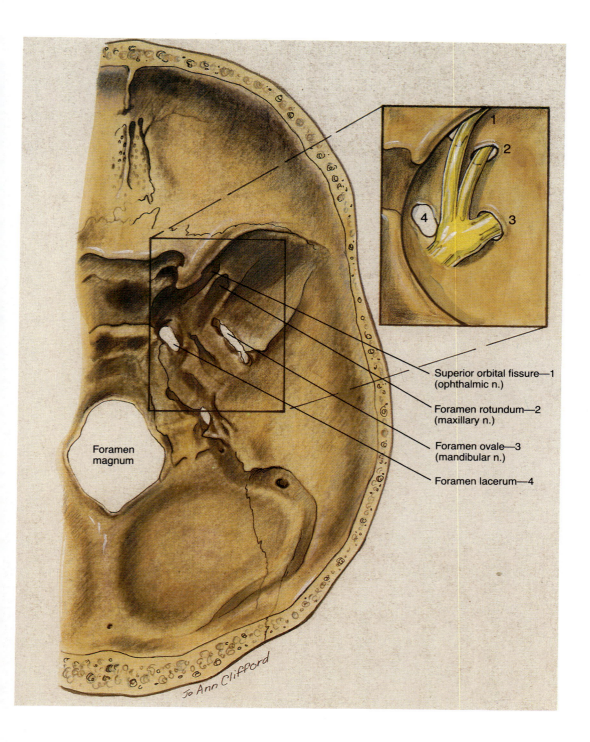

Figure 16–3 Intracranial anatomy—trigeminal nerve and branches

Superior orbital fissure—1
(ophthalmic n.)

Foramen rotundum—2
(maxillary n.)

Foramen ovale—3
(mandibular n.)

Foramen lacerum—4

Foramen
magnum

Jo Ann Clifford

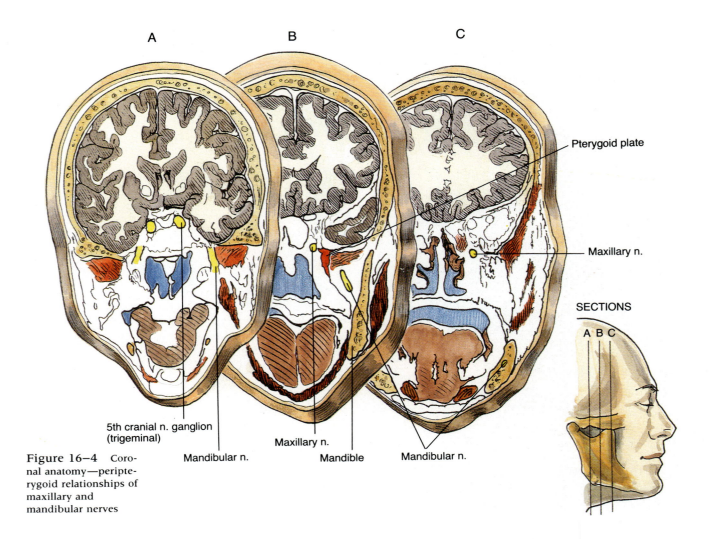

Figure 16–4 Coronal anatomy—pteripterygoid relationships of maxillary and mandibular nerves

A   B   C

Pterygoid plate

Maxillary n.

SECTIONS

A B C

5th cranial n. ganglion
(trigeminal)

Maxillary n.

Mandibular n.

Mandible

Mandibular n.

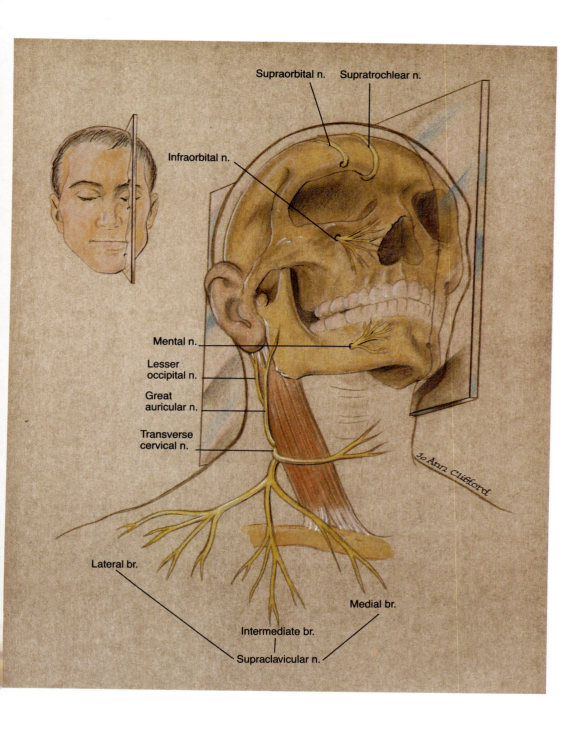

Supraorbital n. Supratrochlear n.

Infraorbital n.

Mental n.

Lesser occipital n.

Great auricular n.

Transverse cervical n.

Lateral br.

Medial br.

Intermediate br.

Supraclavicular n.

Jo Ann Clifford

Figure 16–5 Head and neck anatomy—superficial relationships

17

Occipital Block

Perspective

Occipital nerve block is most frequently used in the diagnosis and treatment of occipital tension headaches. It is also useful when combined with other head and neck blockade to provide scalp anesthesia when infiltration alone will not suffice.

Patient Selection. Most patients for occipital nerve block will be experiencing occipital tension headaches. These patients often will be at the end of a long and frustrating medical program and thus may need detailed explanation of what to expect during blockade.

Pharmacologic Choice. This block requires only 3 to 5 ml of local anesthetic, so virtually any local anesthetic can be utilized.

Placement

Anatomy. The greater occipital nerve arises from the dorsal rami of the second cervical nerve and travels deep to cervical musculature until it becomes subcutaneous slightly inferior to the superior nuchal line. It emerges on this line in association with the occipital artery, and the artery is the most useful landmark for locating the greater occipital nerve (Fig. 17–1).

Position. The most effective patient position for greater occipital blockade is sitting, with the chin flexed upon the chest. A short,

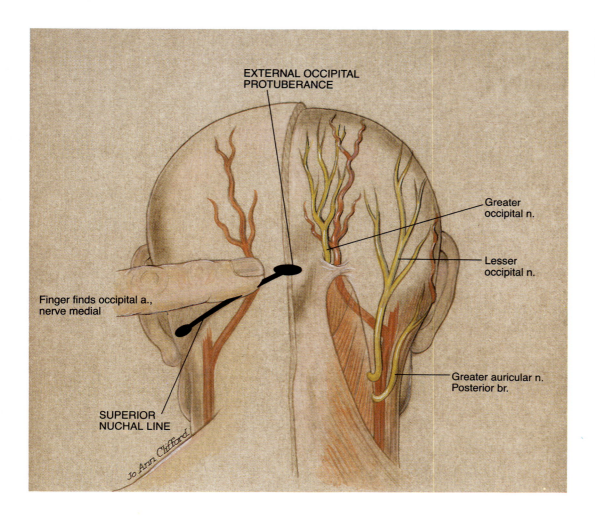

EXTERNAL OCCIPITAL PROTUBERANCE

Greater occipital n.

Lesser occipital n.

Finger finds occipital a., nerve medial

Greater auricular n. Posterior br.

SUPERIOR NUCHAL LINE

Jo Ann Clifford

Figure 17–1 Occipital nerve block— anatomy and technique

25-gauge needle is inserted through the skin at the level of the superior nuchal line so as to develop a "wall" of local anesthetic surrounding the posterior occipital artery. The artery is commonly found approximately one third of the distance between the external occipital protuberance and the mastoid process on the superior nuchal line. Injection of 3 to 5 ml of local anesthetic in this area will produce satisfactory anesthesia.

Potential Problems. The superficial nature of this block should make complications infrequent.

Pearls

To make this block effective for pain diagnosis and therapy, the anesthesiologist must make clear to the patient what the expectations are before performing the block. Often patients reach the anesthesiologist only after a long and arduous trial of alternative pain therapies; thus it is as important for the anesthesiologist to handle the psychosocial implications of the procedure as it is to discuss the technical features.

18

Trigeminal Block

Trigeminal (Gasserian) Ganglion Block

Perspective

Although the trigeminal ganglion block can be used for surgical procedures involving the face, its principal use is as a diagnostic block prior to trigeminal neurolysis in patients with facial neuralgias. Even after the anesthesiologist successfully identifies that the trigeminal nerve is responsible for facial pain, neurolysis is most often carried out today using thermocoagulation techniques rather than neurolytic solutions.

Patient Selection. Current practice patterns virtually guarantee that patients undergoing this block will be experiencing facial neuralgias. It is possible that patients with severe underlying cardiopulmonary disease who require more than minor facial surgery may be candidates for local anesthetic trigeminal ganglion blockade.

Pharmacologic Choice. Trigeminal ganglion block can be carried out with 1 to 3 ml of local anesthetic; thus, almost any of the local anesthetics is an option.

Placement

Anatomy. The trigeminal ganglion is located intracranially and measures approximately 1 × 2 cm. In its intracranial location it lies lateral to the internal carotid artery and cavernous sinus and slightly posterior and superior to the foramen ovale, through which the mandibular nerve leaves the cranium (Fig. 18–1). From the trigeminal ganglion, the fifth cranial nerve divides into its three principal divisions: the ophthalmic, maxillary, and mandibular nerves. These nerves provide sensation to the region of the eye and forehead, upper jaw (midface), and lower jaw, respectively (Fig. 18–1). The mandibular division carries motor fibers to the muscles of mastication, but otherwise these nerves are wholly sensory. The trigeminal ganglion is partially contained within a reflection of dura mater, Meckel's cave. Figures 18–2 and 3 show that the foramen ovale is approximately in the horizontal plane of the zygoma and in the frontal plane approximately at the level of the mandibular notch. The foramen ovale is slightly less than 1 cm in diameter and

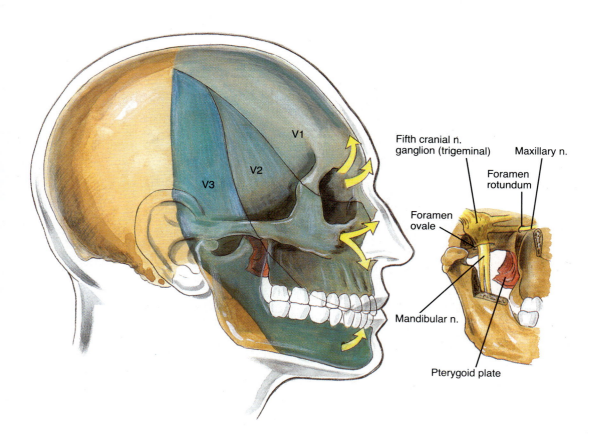

Figure 18–1 Fifth cranial nerve ganglion (trigeminal) anatomy—innervation and peripterygoid relationships

V1

V2

V3

Fifth cranial n. ganglion (trigeminal)

Maxillary n.

Foramen rotundum

Foramen ovale

Mandibular n.

Pterygoid plate

Figure 18–2 Cross-sectional anatomy—fifth cranial nerve (trigeminal) ganglion and foramen ovale

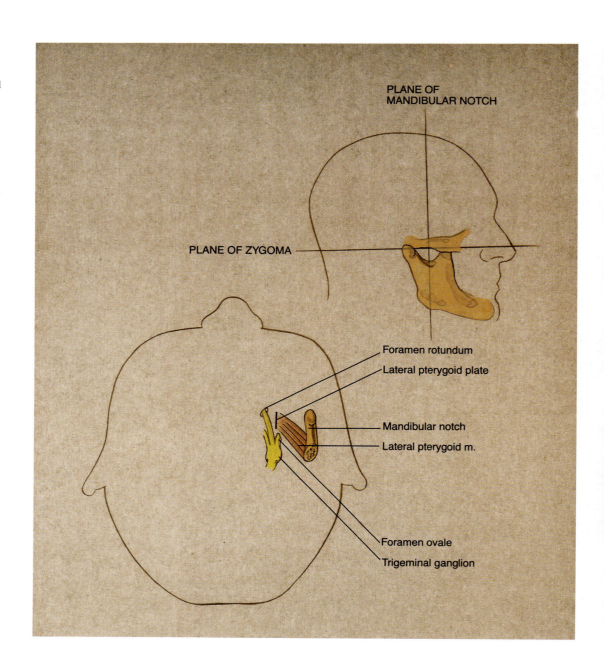

PLANE OF
MANDIBULAR NOTCH

PLANE OF ZYGOMA

Foramen rotundum

Lateral pterygoid plate

Mandibular notch

Lateral pterygoid m.

Foramen ovale

Trigeminal ganglion

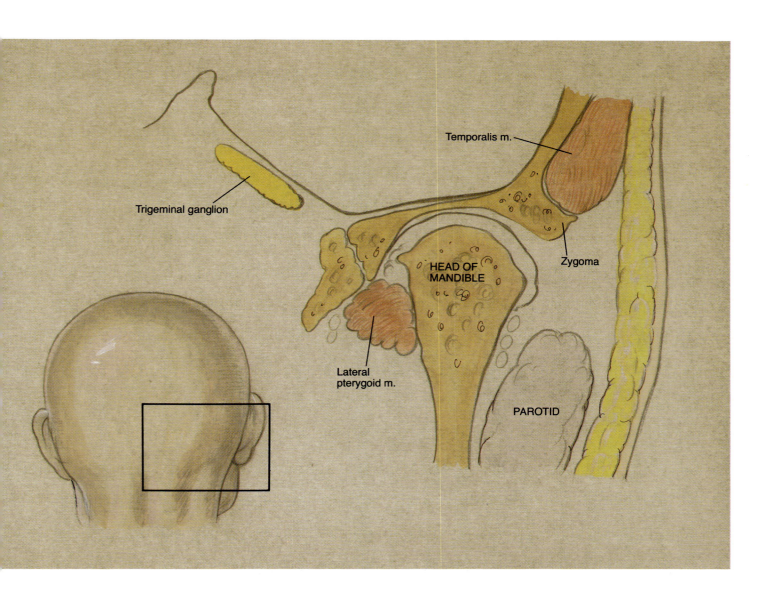

Trigeminal ganglion

Temporalis m.

Zygoma

HEAD OF MANDIBLE

Lateral pterygoid m.

PAROTID

Figure 18–3 Coronal anatomy—section through fifth cranial nerve (trigeminal) ganglion

Figure 18—4 Trigeminal ganglion block—anatomy and needle insertion plane

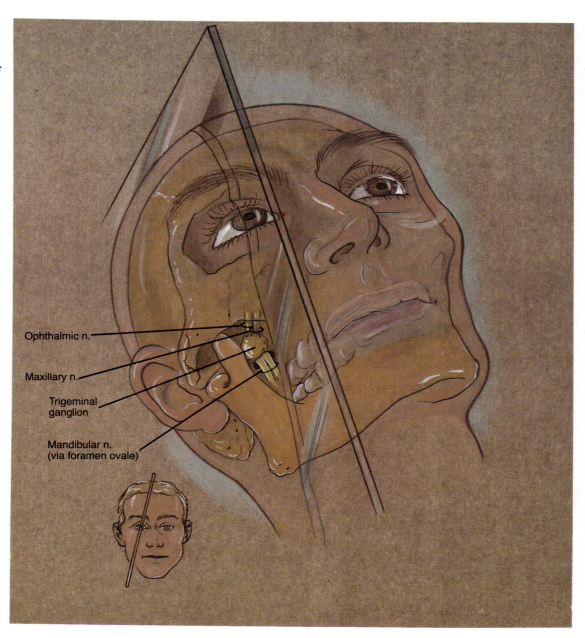

Ophthalmic n.

Maxillary n.

Trigeminal ganglion

Mandibular n. (via foramen ovale)

is situated immediately dorsolateral to the pterygoid process.

Position. Patients are placed in a supine position and asked to fix their gaze straight ahead, as if they were looking off into the distance. The anesthesiologist should be positioned at the patient's side, slightly below the level of the shoulder, so that by looking toward the patient's face the perspective shown in Figure 18—4 is observed.

Needle Puncture. A skin wheal is raised immediately medial to the masseter muscle, which can be located by asking the patient to clench the teeth. (It will most often occur approximately 3 cm lateral to the corner of the mouth.) Through this site, as illustrated in Figure 18—5, a 22-gauge, 10-cm needle is inserted as at position 1. The plane of insertion should be in line with the pupil, as illustrated in Figure 18—4. This will allow the needle tip

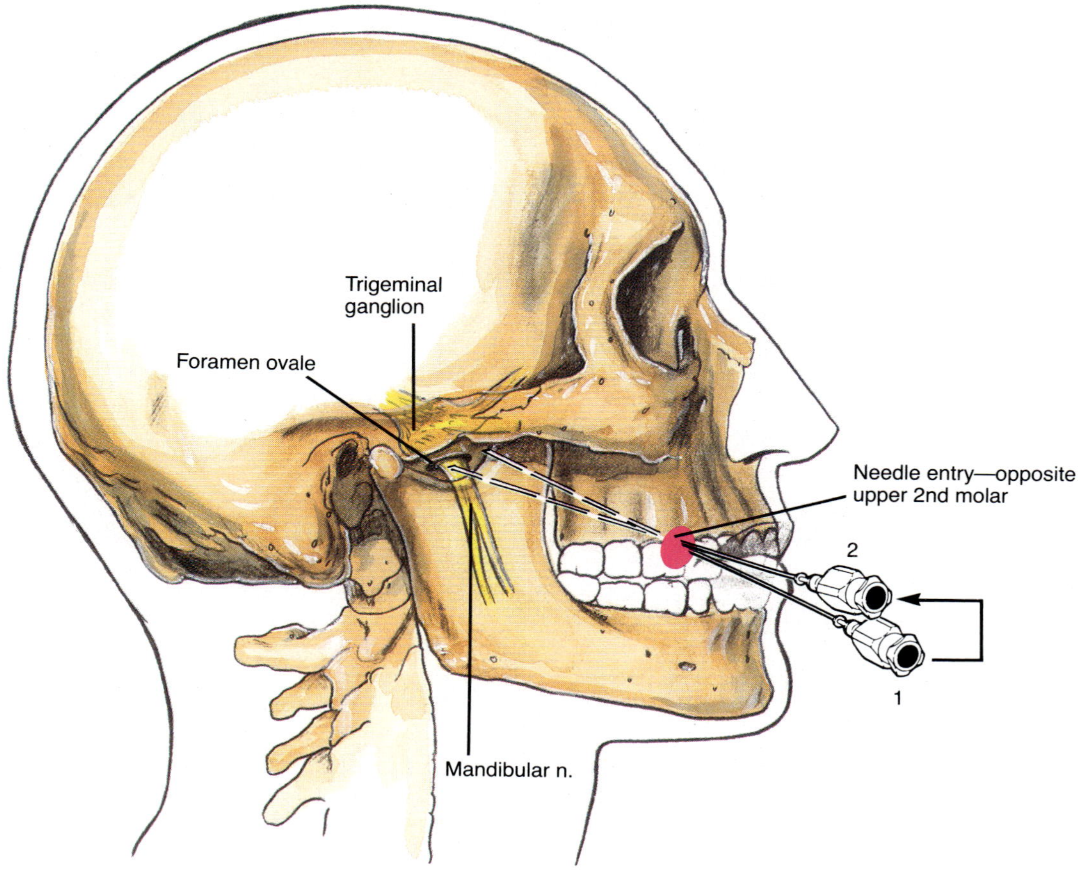
Trigeminal ganglion
Foramen ovale
Needle entry—opposite upper 2nd molar
2
1
Mandibular n.

Figure 18–5 Trigeminal ganglion block—anatomy and technique

to contact the infratemporal surface of the greater wing of the sphenoid bone, immediately anterior to the foramen ovale. This occurs at a depth of from 4.5 to 6 cm. Once the needle is firmly positioned against this infratemporal region, it is withdrawn and redirected in a step-wise manner until it enters the foramen ovale at a depth of approximately 6 to 7 cm, or 1 to 1.5 cm past the needle length required to contact the bone initially.

As the foramen is entered, a mandibular paresthesia is often elicited. By advancing the needle slightly, one may also elicit paresthesia in the distribution of the ophthalmic or maxillary nerves. These additional paresthesias should be sought in order to verify a periganglion position of the needle tip. If the only paresthesia obtained is in the mandibular distribution, the needle tip may not have entered the foramen ovale but rather be inferior to it while it abuts the mandibular nerve.

Prior to injection of local anesthetic, careful aspiration of the needle should be performed to check for cerebrospinal fluid (CSF), since the ganglion's posterior two thirds is enveloped in the reflection of dura, Meckel's cave. If trigeminal block is being undertaken diagnostically prior to neurolysis, 1 ml of local anesthetic should now be injected. Nerve blockade should develop within 5 to 10 minutes, and, if blockade is incomplete, an additional 1 to 2 ml of local anesthetic can be injected, or the needle can be repositioned in an effort to obtain a more complete blockade.

Potential Problems. It is obvious that subarachnoid injection of local anesthetic is possible with this block, owing to the close anatomic relationship between the trigeminal ganglion and the dural reflection, Meckel's cave. Likewise, the needle will pass through highly vascular regions on its way to the foramen ovale, and hematoma formation is a possibility. The block can also be painful for the patient and may require effective sedation prior to final needle placement.

Pearls

As with all regional block techniques, it is important not to develop a sense of "time pressure" when performing this block. This is especially pertinent to trigeminal ganglion block, since doses of 1% lidocaine as small as 0.25 ml have produced unconsciousness when unintentionally injected into the CSF during the block. Since this block can be uncomfortable, sufficient time is needed to allow for appropriate sedation and for the patient to become comfortable with the approach.

19

Maxillary Block

Perspective

Local anesthetic blockade of the maxillary nerve in its peripterygoid location is most commonly used to evaluate facial neuralgia. However, it can be used to facilitate surgical procedures in its cutaneous distribution (Fig. 19–1). Injection of neurolytic solution from the lateral approach to the maxillary nerve in its peripterygoid location should be undertaken with extreme caution owing to its location near the orbit.

Patient Selection. This block will principally be used diagnostically in the workup of facial neuralgia. For patients with significant cardiopulmonary disease who require a surgical procedure in the distribution of the maxillary nerve, it can be utilized for surgical anesthesia.

Pharmacologic Choice. The maxillary nerve can be blocked with a low volume of local anesthetic (less than 5 ml); thus, virtually any local anesthetic can be chosen.

Placement

Anatomy. The maxillary nerve is entirely sensory and passes through the foramen rotundum to exit from the cranium. The nerve passes through the pterygopalatine fossa, medial to the lateral pterygoid plate on its way to enter the infraorbital fissure. As illustrated in Figure 19–2, it is accessible to the anesthesiologist via a lateral approach as it passes into the pterygopalatine fossa.

Position. The patient is placed in the supine position with the head and neck rotated away from the side to be blocked. While the anesthesiologist palpates the mandibular notch, the patient is asked to open and close the mouth gently to make the notch even more obvious.

Needle Puncture. A 22-gauge, 8-cm needle is inserted through the mandibular notch in a slightly cephalomedial direction, as illustrated in Figure 19–3. This allows the needle to impinge upon the lateral pterygoid plate at

Figure 19–1 Maxillary nerve (V$_2$) cutaneous innervation

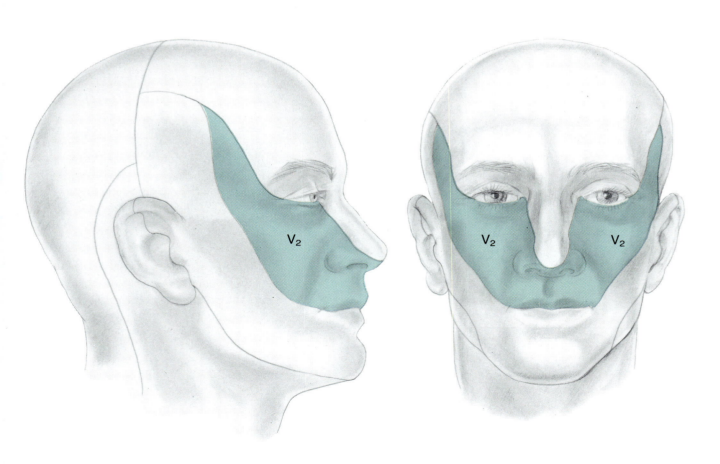

Figure 19–2 Maxillary block anatomy—peripterygoid relationships

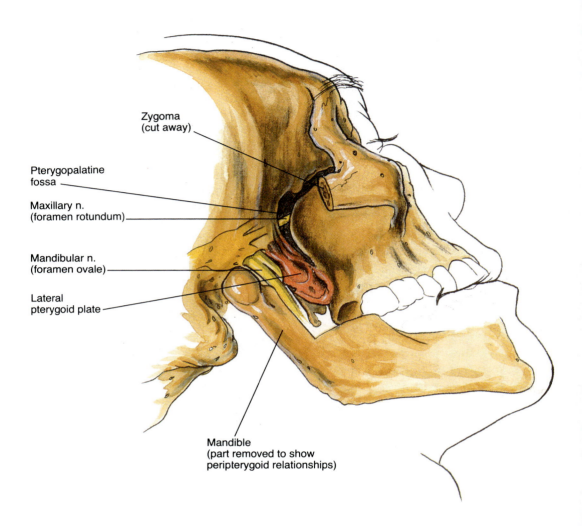

Zygoma
(cut away)

Pterygopalatine
fossa

Maxillary n.
(foramen rotundum)

Mandibular n.
(foramen ovale)

Lateral
pterygoid plate

Mandible
(part removed to show
peripterygoid relationships)

a depth of approximately 5 cm (needle position 1). The needle is then withdrawn and redirected in a step-wise manner toward position 2 (the pterygopalatine fossa). The needle should not be advanced more than 1 cm past the depth of initial contact with the pterygoid plate. As the needle is walked off the pterygoid plate, a "sense" of walking into the pterygopalatine fossa should be appreciated. Once the needle is adequately positioned, 5 ml of local anesthetic is injected.

Potential Problems. Due to the close association of the maxillary nerve to the infraorbital fissure, some spill of local anesthetic into the orbit is possible; thus, patients should be warned that movement of the eye and/or vision might be affected. The lateral approach

to the maxillary nerve also involves insertion of the needle through a vascular region, and hematoma formation is possible. Again, due to the close association of the pterygopalatine fossa to the orbit, patients frequently develop a "black eye" following this block.

Pearls

To be comfortable and clinically successful with this block, anesthesiologists should find the time to examine the relationship of the foramen rotundum, pterygoid plate, and pterygopalatine fossa. An understanding of the peripterygoid anatomy will promote an anesthesiologist's confidence and the clinical efficacy of this block.

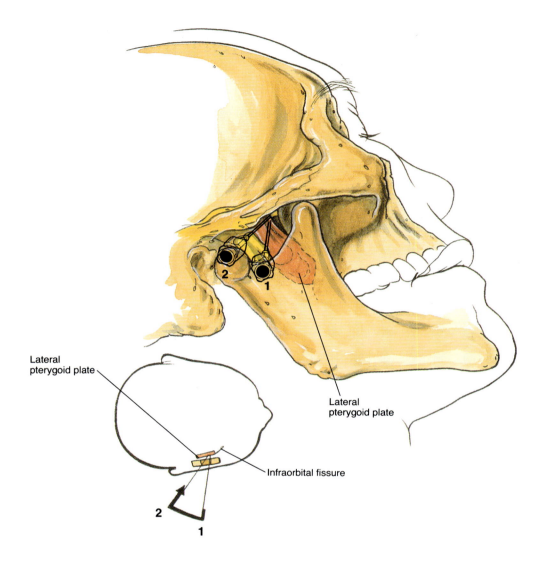

Lateral
pterygoid plate

Lateral
pterygoid plate

Infraorbital fissure

Figure 19–3 Maxillary block anatomy—needle insertion technique

Perspective

This block is most often used for diagnosis of facial neuralgias; however, it can be used for surgical procedures upon the skin overlying the lower jaw, except at the jaw's angle. Dental procedures upon the lower jaw can also be carried out, although the intraoral approach to the mandibular nerve is more commonly performed by dentists for the block.

Patient Selection. Patients appropriate for this block are those with facial neuralgias and those with significant cardiopulmonary disease who require a surgical procedure in the region innervated by mandibular nerve blockade.

Pharmacologic Choice. Since small volumes (5 ml) of local anesthetic will produce regional blockade of the mandibular nerve, virtually any local anesthetic agent is an acceptable choice.

Placement

Anatomy. The mandibular nerve is a mixed motor sensory nerve, although primarily sensory. It exits from the cranium through the foramen ovale and parallels the posterior margin of the lateral pterygoid plate as it descends inferiorly and laterally toward the mandible (Figs. 20–1 and 20–2). The anterior division of the mandibular nerve is principally motor and supplies the muscles of mastication, whereas the posterior division is principally sensory and supplies the skin and mucous membranes overlying the lower jaw and skin anterior and superior to the ear (Fig. 20–3). Sensory branches of the man-

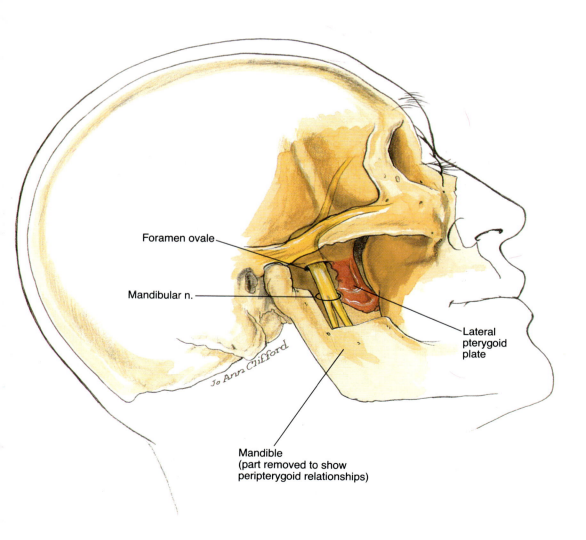

Figure 20–1 Mandibular block anatomy—peripterygoid relationships

Foramen ovale

Mandibular n.

Lateral pterygoid plate

Jo Ann Clifford

Mandible (part removed to show peripterygoid relationships)

Figure 20-2 Coronal anatomy—peripterygoid relationships

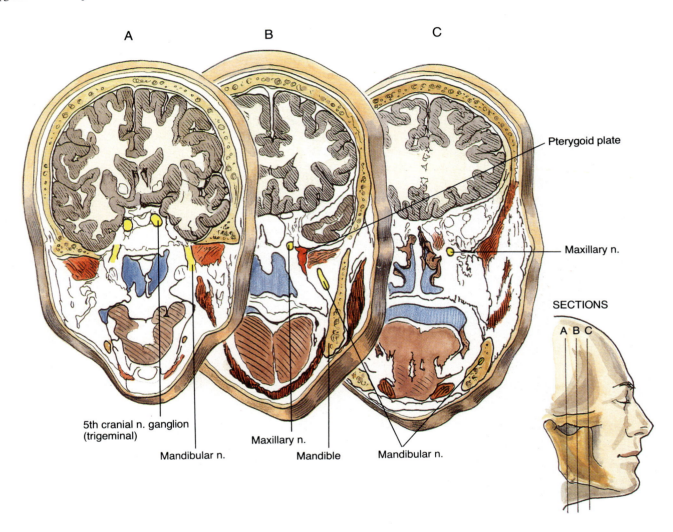

Pterygoid plate

Maxillary n.

SECTIONS

A B C

5th cranial n. ganglion (trigeminal)

Mandibular n.

Maxillary n.

Mandible

Mandibular n.

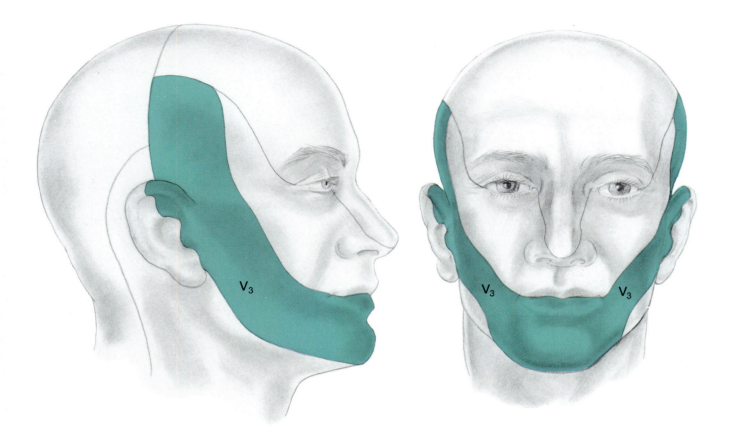

Figure 20–3 Mandibular nerve (V₃) cutaneous innervation

dibular nerve are buccal, auriculotemporal, lingual, and inferior alveolar nerves. The *buccal nerve* is exclusively sensory and supplies the mucous membranes of the cheek. The *auriculotemporal nerve* passes posterior to the neck of the mandible to supply skin anterior to the ear and into the scalp's temporal region. The *lingual nerve* is joined by the chorda tympani branch of the facial nerve, and together they supply taste and general sensation to the anterior two thirds of the tongue and sensation to the floor of the mouth, including the lingual aspect of the lower gingivae. The *inferior alveolar nerve* supplies the lower teeth and terminates as the mental nerve, which supplies sensation to the lower labial mucous membranes and skin of the chin.

Position. The patient is placed in the supine position, with the head and neck turned away from the side to be blocked. As in the approach used for maxillary blockade, the patient is asked to open and close the mouth gently while the anesthesiologist palpates the mandibular notch to identify it more clearly.

Needle Puncture. The needle is inserted in the mid point of the mandibular notch and directed to reach the lateral pterygoid plate by taking a slightly cephalomedial angle through the notch, as shown in Figure 20–4. The 22-gauge, 8-cm needle will impinge on the lateral pterygoid plate at a depth of approximately 5 cm (needle position 1). The needle is then withdrawn and redirected in small steps to walk off the posterior border of the lateral pterygoid plate in a horizontal plane, as shown in Figure 20–4. The needle should not be advanced more than 0.5 cm past the depth of the pterygoid plate, because the superior constrictor muscle of the pharynx is easily pierced; thus, the pharynx will be entered if the needle is inserted more

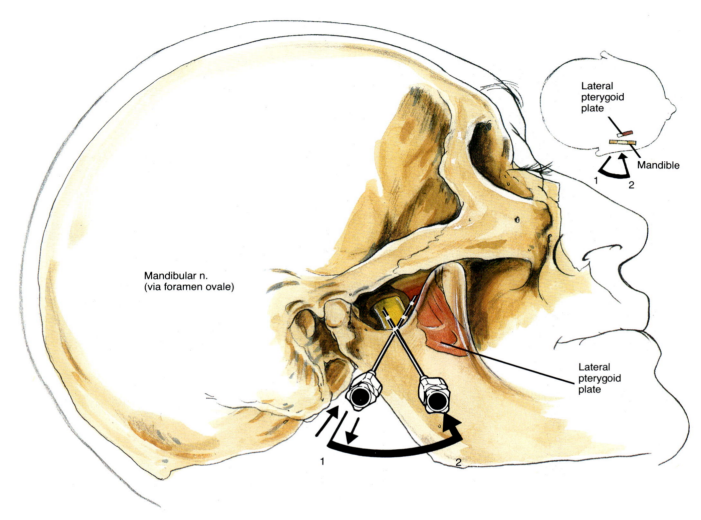

Lateral
pterygoid
plate

Mandible

1

2

Mandibular n.
(via foramen ovale)

Lateral
pterygoid
plate

1

2

Figure 20–4 Mandibular block anatomy—needle insertion technique

deeply. Once the needle tip is appropriately positioned, 5 ml of local anesthetic is administered.

Potential Problems. As with maxillary nerve blockade, the lateral approach to the mandibular nerve requires needle insertion through a vascular region. Thus, hematoma formation is possible. If a hematoma does occur, most often watchful waiting is all that is required. In spite of greater difficulty entering the cerebrospinal fluid (CSF) through the foramen ovale from the lateral approach, one needs to be constantly aware that if a needle is inserted via the foramen ovale into Meckel's cave, small doses of local anesthetic in the CSF can produce unconsciousness.

Pearls

As with maxillary nerve block, anesthesiologists should develop a thorough understanding of peripterygoid anatomy prior to carrying out this block. Needle movements with the mandibular block involve fewer "planes" than with maxillary block, since the needle is moved primarily in the horizontal plane once the pterygoid plate is contacted. Therefore, in some ways, it is less complex than the maxillary block. Also, since the mandibular nerve is more distant from orbital structures, one does not have to be as worried about using neurolytic solutions with this block.

21

Distal Trigeminal Block

Perspective

This block can be used for the diagnosis of facial neuralgia; however, more frequently it is utilized for superficial surgical procedures that require more than simple infiltration for anesthesia.

Patient Selection. Almost all patients are candidates for distal trigeminal blockade, since the bony foramina—supraorbital, infraorbital, and mental—are easily palpable.

Pharmacologic Choice. Owing to the small volumes of local anesthetic necessary for this block, almost any local anesthetic agent may be chosen.

Placement

Anatomy. The distal branches of the three divisions of the trigeminal nerve—ophthalmic (supraorbital), maxillary (infraorbital), and mandibular (mental)—exit from the skull through their respective foramina on a line that runs almost vertically through the pupil (Fig. 21–1).

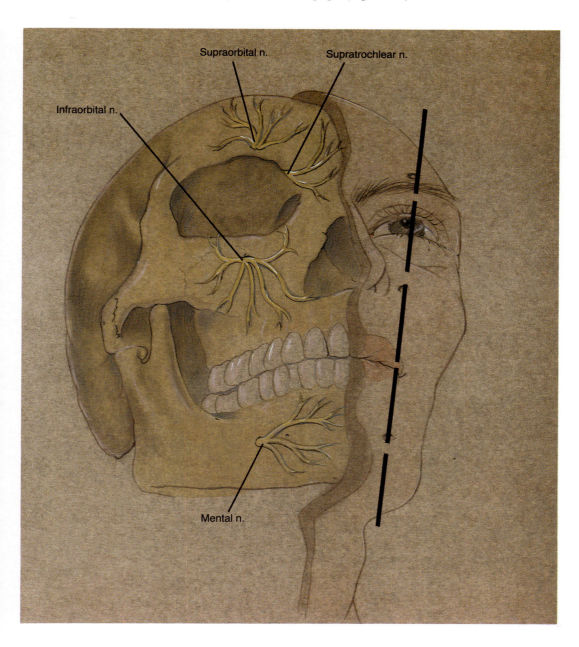

Supraorbital n.

Supratrochlear n.

Infraorbital n.

Mental n.

Figure 21–1 Distal trigeminal anatomy

Position. The patient is placed in the supine position with the anesthesiologist at the patient's side, approximately at the level of the shoulder.

Needle Puncture. For this block, as illustrated in Figure 21–2, once the respective foramina are identified by palpation, a short, 25-gauge needle is inserted in a cephalomedial direction, and approximately 2 to 3 ml of local anesthetic is injected at the site. If a paresthesia is obtained, the local anesthetic can be deposited at that point.

Potential Problems. This block is superficial and thus carries with it few complications.

One should be cautious about entering the foramina to inject the local anesthetic, since intraneural injection is probably more frequent with that approach.

Pearls

The anesthesiologist should assure that the patient is properly sedated and should clearly identify the foramina to be blocked, so that accurate needle placement is achieved.

Figure 21–2 Distal trigeminal block—technique

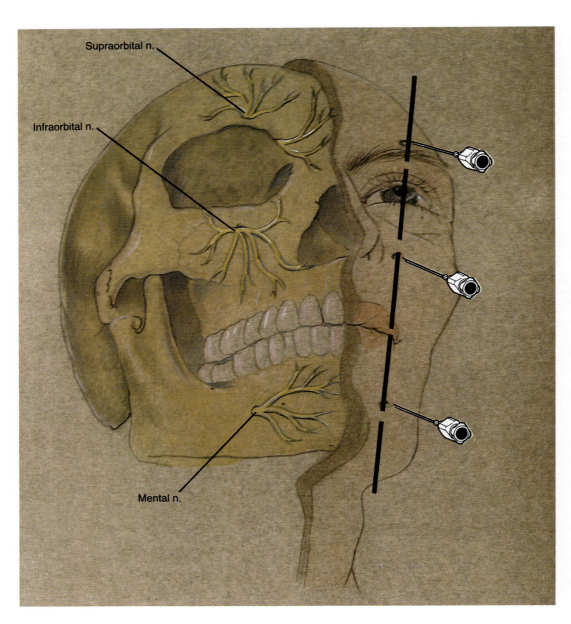

22

Retrobulbar (Peribulbar) Block

Perspective

Many anesthesiologists do not commonly carry out this block; rather, most often oph-thalmologists utilize this very useful applica-tion of regional blockade. The combination of retrobulbar anesthesia and block of the or-bicularis oculi muscle allows most intraocular surgery to be performed. This regional block is most useful for corneal, anterior chamber, and lens procedures.

Patient Selection. The patients who require retrobulbar (peribulbar) anesthesia are princi-pally older patients who are undergoing oph-thalmic operations.

Pharmacologic Choice. If retrobulbar block is used, 2 to 4 ml of local anesthetic is all that is required to produce adequate retro-bulbar anesthesia. Conversely, if the peribul-bar approach is chosen (that is, the needle tip is not purposely inserted through the cone of extraocular muscles), slightly larger volumes, 4 to 6 ml, may be necessary. Once again, almost any of the local anesthetic agents are applicable, with many ophthalmo-logic anesthetists utilizing combinations of bupivacaine and lidocaine.

Placement

Anatomy. Sensation to the eye is provided by the ophthalmic nerve, via the long and short posterior ciliary nerves. Autonomic in-nervation is provided by these same nerves, while sympathetic fibers traveling with the arteries and parasympathetic fibers carried by the inferior branch of the oculomotor nerve provide additional autonomic innervation. Because the innervation of the orbicularis oculi muscle is via the facial nerve, blockade of these fibers is required to ensure a quiet eye during ophthalmic operation. The ciliary ganglion, measuring approximately 2 to 3 mm in length, lies deep within the orbit just lateral to the optic nerve and medial to the

Figure 22−1 Orbit-al anatomy

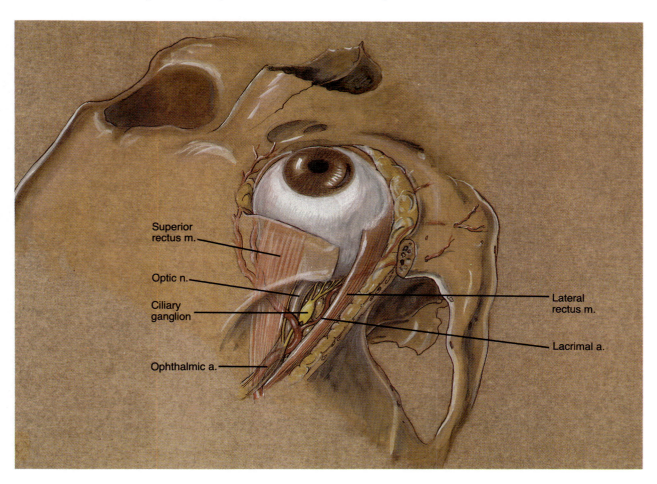

Superior rectus m.

Optic n.

Ciliary ganglion

Ophthalmic a.

Lateral rectus m.

Lacrimal a.

lateral rectus muscle. From this ganglion the long and short ciliary nerves extend forward in the orbit. Immediately posterior to the ciliary ganglion, the ophthalmic artery can be found at the lateral side of the optic nerve as it crosses superior to it and passes forward in a medial direction (Fig. 22–1).

Position. Patients are placed in the supine position and are instructed to look opposite the site of injection and slightly cephalad. The anesthesiologist is positioned for the injection as illustrated in Figure 22–2.

Needle puncture. While the patient is looking cephalad and opposite the site of injection, a 23- to 25-gauge, 3.5-cm-long, short-beveled needle is inserted at the inferolateral border of the bony orbit and directed toward the apex of the orbit, as illustrated in Figure 22–3. A "pop" is often appreciated as the needle tip traverses the bulbar fascia and enters the orbital muscle cone. Prior to injecting

2 to 4 ml of local anesthetic, careful aspiration of the needle should be carried out. Following retrobulbar block, 5 to 10 minutes should be allowed to pass before the operation is started. This helps avoid operating on patients who develop retrobulbar hematomas. During these 5 to 10 minutes, the anesthesiologist can apply gentle pressure to the globe, principally to facilitate lowering of intraocular pressure. If a peribulbar technique is chosen, needle insertion begins like that for retrobulbar injection; however, the needle is inserted parallel and lateral to the lateral rectus muscle and bulbar fascia rather than making an effort to puncture it. To complete the local block for ocular surgery, the orbicularis oculi muscle must be blocked to produce an immobile eye. This is carried out by blocking the facial nerve fibers that innervate the muscle.

There are many ways of performing blocks

Figure 22–2 Retrobulbar (peribulbar) block—technique

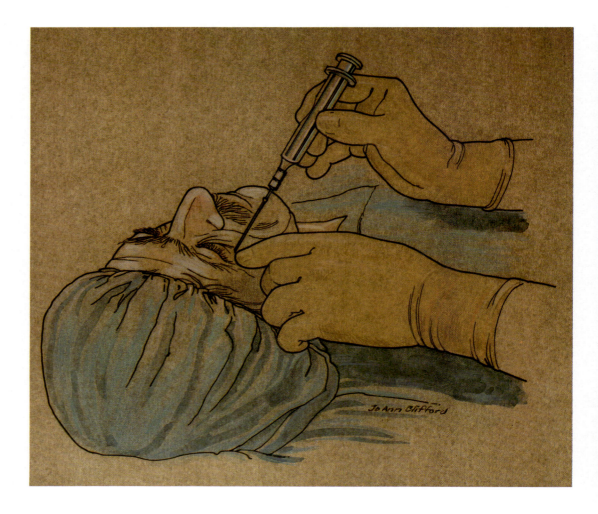

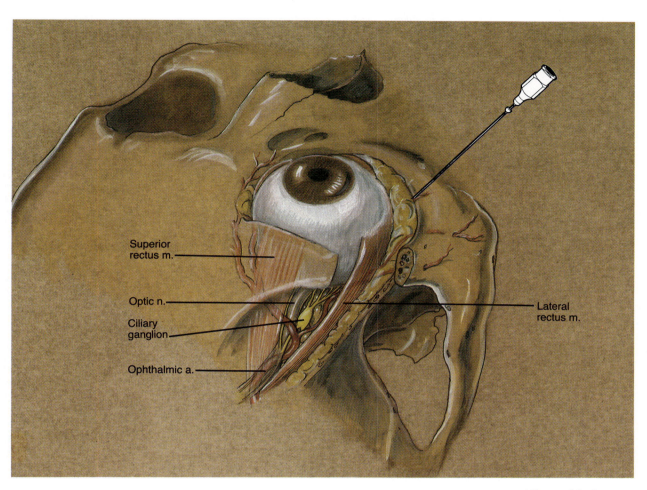

Superior rectus m.

Optic n.

Ciliary ganglion

Ophthalmic a.

Lateral rectus m.

Figure 22–3 Retrobulbar (peribulbar) block—technique

of these facial nerve fibers, and the method illustrated in Figure 22–4 is the example of Van Lint. In this block, a 25-gauge, 4-cm needle is inserted at needle position 1 until the lower inferolateral orbital rim is reached. While the needle tip contacts bony surface, 1 ml of local anesthetic is injected. Through this skin wheal, the needle is repositioned along the lateral and inferior margins of the orbit (needle positions 2 and 3), and 2 to 3 ml of local anesthetic is injected along each needle path.

Potential Problems. The most common complication that accompanies retrobulbar block is hematoma formation. This can be minimized by using a needle shorter than 3.5 cm, which also has a blunt tip. Hematoma formation is more likely if a longer needle is used and the needle tip rests in the vicinity of the ophthalmic artery as it crosses the optic nerve. As outlined, this can also be avoided by utilizing a peribulbar approach. Other complications that can accompany retrobulbar block include local anesthetic toxicity, development of the oculocardiac reflex,

and cases of sudden apnea and obtundation following retrobulbar injection. The latter two are probably related to injection within the optic nerve sheath, resulting in unexpected spinal anesthesia, or intravascular injection affecting respiratory centers in the midbrain, as illustrated in Figure 22–5.

Pearls

If anesthesiologists carry out retrobulbar anesthesia, they must work with ophthalmologists who are supportive and willing to share this part of their practice. Many of the complications of retrobulbar anesthesia can be avoided if peribulbar block is carried out. Once again, this can be produced by placing the needle along the muscular cone of extraocular muscles, rather than within the muscular cone. Slightly larger volumes of local anesthetic are required; however, most of the major complications can be avoided in this fashion.

Figure 22–4 Regional block of orbicularis oculi muscle— Van Lint method

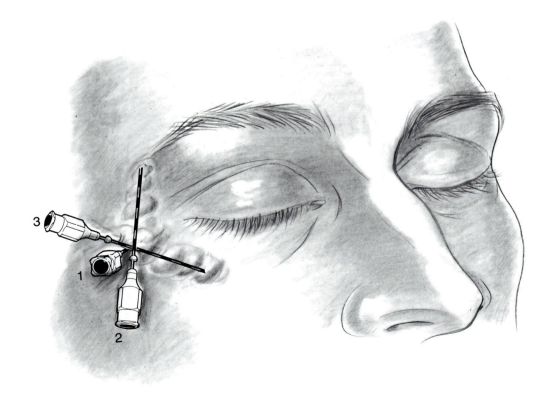

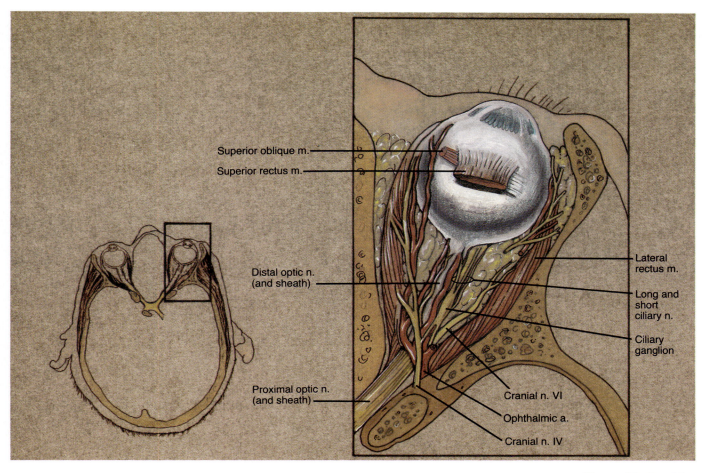

Superior oblique m.

Superior rectus m.

Distal optic n.
(and sheath)

Proximal optic n.
(and sheath)

Lateral
rectus m.

Long and
short
ciliary n.

Ciliary
ganglion

Cranial n. VI

Ophthalmic a.

Cranial n. IV

Figure 22–5 Orbital functional anatomy

23

Cervical Plexus Block

Perspective

Cervical plexus blockade can be utilized to carry out both superficial and deep operations within the region of the neck and supraclavicular fossa. The choice of deep or superficial block requires consideration of the surgical procedure.

Patient Selection. This block can be performed easily in a supine patient; thus almost any patient is a candidate for blockade. Bilateral deep cervical plexus block should be avoided, since the phrenic nerve may be partially blocked with the technique. Examples of procedures that are suitable for this technique are carotid endarterectomy, lymph node biopsy, and plastic surgical procedures.

Pharmacologic Choice. Most procedures that are carried out with cervical plexus block do not demand significant motor relaxation. Thus, lower concentrations of local anesthetics, such as 0.75% to 1% lidocaine or mepivacaine, or 0.25% bupivacaine, are appropriate with these techniques.

Placement

Anatomy. Cervical plexus block can be divided into superficial and deep techniques. The cutaneous innervation of the cervical nerves is schematically illustrated in Figure 23–1. The cervical nerves have both dorsal and ventral rami, and those illustrated in Figure 23–2 represent the ventral rami of C1–4. Additionally, there are both sensory and mo-

Figure 23–1 Cervical plexus anatomy—cutaneous innervation

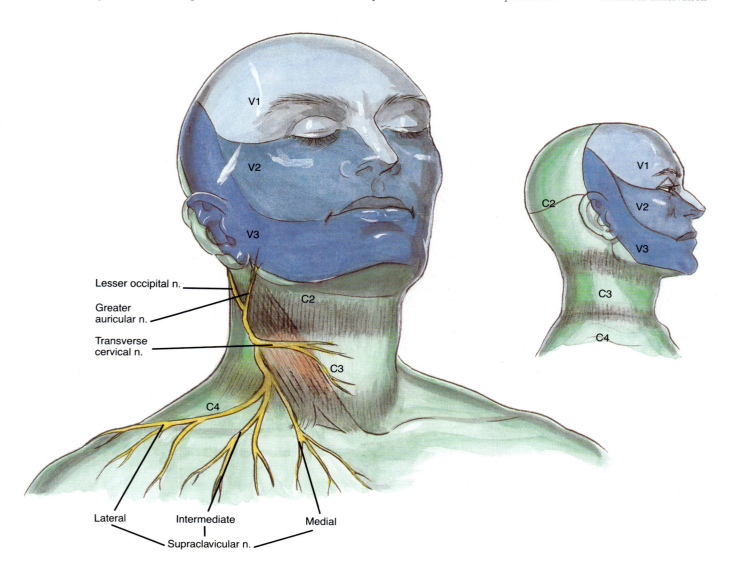

Figure 23-2 Cervical plexus functional anatomy—ventral rami of C1, 2, 3, 4

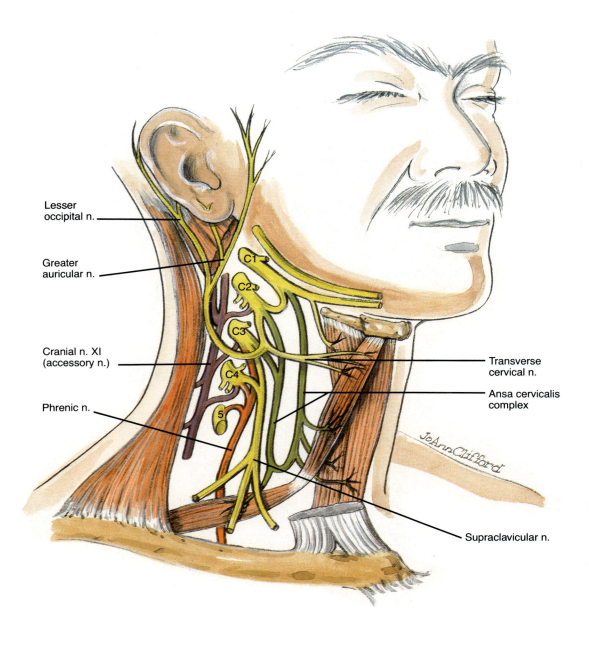

Lesser occipital n.

Greater auricular n.

C1

C2

C3

Cranial n. XI (accessory n.)

C4

Phrenic n.

5

Transverse cervical n.

Ansa cervicalis complex

Supraclavicular n.

JoAnnClifford

tor branches from the dorsal rami of C1–4 that are not shown. Prior to regrouping to form the cervical plexus, the cervical nerves exit from the cervical vertebrae through a gutter in the transverse process in an antero-caudal-lateral direction, immediately posterior to the vertebral artery.

To simplify understanding of the cervical plexus, it can be divided into (1) cutaneous branches of the plexus, (2) the ansa cervicalis complex, (3) the phrenic nerve, (4) contributions to the accessory nerve, and (5) direct muscular branches (Fig. 23–2). The cutaneous branches of the plexus are the lesser occipital, greater auricular, transverse cervical, and supraclavicular nerves (see Fig. 23–1). The first three arise from the second and third cervical nerves, while the supraclavicular nerves arise from the third and fourth cervical nerves. The *ansa cervicalis complex* provides innervation to the infrahyoid and geniohyoid muscles. The *phrenic nerve* is the sole motor nerve to the diaphragm and also provides sensation to its central portion. The nerve arises by a large root from the fourth cervical nerve, reinforced by smaller contributions from the third and fifth nerves. Its course takes it to the lateral border of the anterior scalene muscle, before it descends vertically over the ventral surface of this muscle and enters the chest along its medial border. The *accessory nerve* (cranial nerve 11) receives contributions from the cervical plexus at several points and provides innervation to the sternocleidomastoid muscle as well as the trapezius muscles. The *direct muscular branches* of the plexus supply prevertebral muscles in the neck. The superficial plexus becomes subcutaneous at the midpoint of the posterior border of the sternocleidomastoid muscle (Fig. 23–3 and see Fig. 23–5).

Position. The patient is placed in the supine position, with the head and neck turned opposite the side to be blocked. The anesthesiologist should stand at the patient's side approximately shoulder high.

Needle Puncture—Deep Cervical Plexus Block. The patient should be positioned with the neck slightly extended and the head turned away from the side to be blocked. A line should be drawn between the tip of the mastoid process and Chassaignac's tubercle (i.e., the most easily palpable transverse process of the cervical vertebra-C6). A second line should be drawn parallel and 1 cm posterior to the first line, as illustrated in Figure 23–4. The C4 transverse process should be located by first finding the C2 transverse process 1 to 2 cm caudal to the mastoid process and then identifying C3 and subsequently C4. These transverse processes are each palpable approximately 1.5 cm caudal to the immediately more cephalad process. Once the C4 transverse process is identified, a 22-gauge, 5-cm needle is inserted immediately over the C4 transverse process so that it will contact that

Figure 23–3 Cervical plexus cross-sectional anatomy—midpoint of sternocleidomastoid muscle

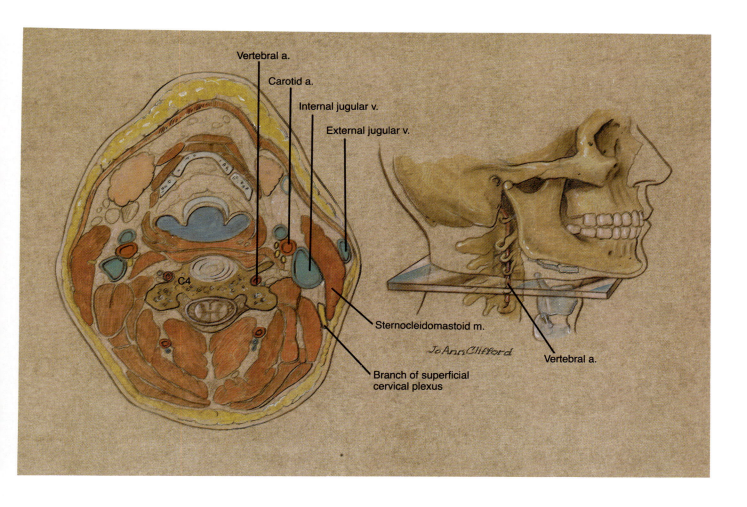

Vertebral a.

Carotid a.

Internal jugular v.

External jugular v.

C4

Sternocleidomastoid m.

Vertebral a.

Branch of superficial cervical plexus

JoAnnClifford

Figure 23–4 Deep cervical plexus block—technique

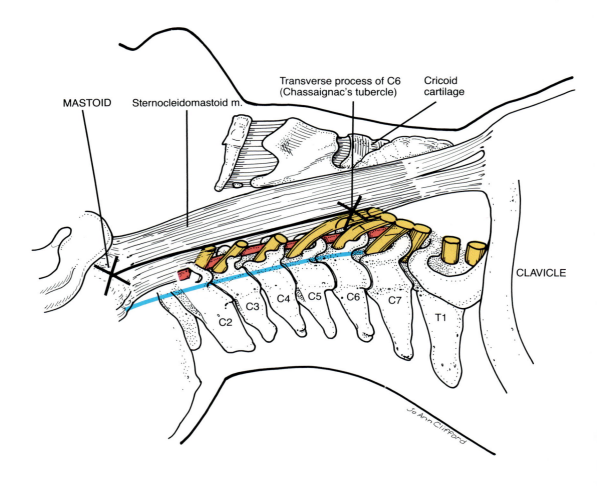

MASTOID

Sternocleidomastoid m.

Transverse process of C6 (Chassaignac's tubercle)

Cricoid cartilage

CLAVICLE

C2 C3 C4 C5 C6 C7 T1

process at a depth of approximately 1.5 to 3 cm. If a paresthesia is obtained, 10 to 12 ml of local anesthetic is injected at this site. It is helpful to obtain a paresthesia with this technique prior to injection since one is relying on continuity of the paravertebral space in the neck to facilitate local anesthetic spread. If a paresthesia is not elicited on the first pass, the needle should be withdrawn and walked in a step-wise fashion in an anterior-posterior manner.

Needle Placement—Superficial Cervical Block.

The superficial cervical plexus block, as illustrated in Figure 23–5, relies on local anesthetic "volume" to be effective. At the midpoint on the posterior border of the sternocleidomastoid muscle, the superficial cervical plexus is packaged so that infiltration deep to the posterior border of the sternocleidomastoid muscle will produce blockade. To perform the block, a 22-gauge, 4-cm needle is inserted subcutaneously posterior and immediately deep to the sternocleidomastoid muscle, and 5 ml of local anesthetic is injected.

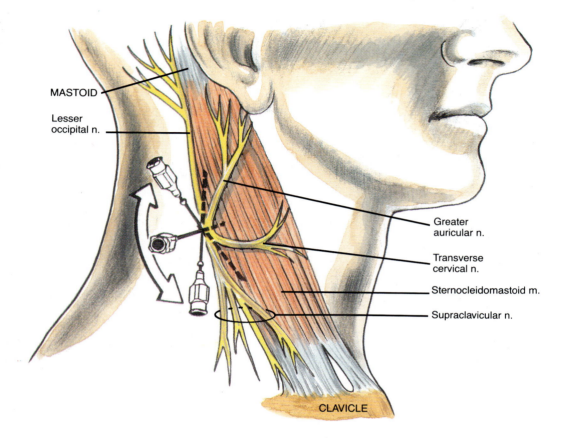

MASTOID

Lesser
occipital n.

Greater
auricular n.

Transverse
cervical n.

Sternocleidomastoid m.

Supraclavicular n.

CLAVICLE

Figure 23–5 Superficial cervical plexus block—anatomy and technique

The needle is then redirected both superiorly and inferiorly along the posterior border of the sternocleidomastoid, with 5 ml of solution injected along each of these sites. In this fashion a field block of the superficial plexus results.

Potential Problems. With deep cervical plexus block, blockade is often accompanied by at least partial phrenic nerve block, and bilateral blocks, therefore, should be used with caution. The block also places the needles near the vertebral artery and other centroneuraxis structures. When carrying out the superficial block, the external jugular vein often overlies the block site and should simply be avoided. Likewise, intravascular injection via the internal jugular vein can occur if the needle is inserted too deeply while the field block is being performed.

Pearls

If patients are properly positioned for this block, the superficial block should rarely result in problems. If the deep block is carried out and proper palpation is used to limit the amount of tissue between the anesthesiologist's fingertips and the transverse process, very short needles can help minimize errant, deep injections. If deep cervical plexus block is to be carried out for carotid endarterectomy, the surgical colleagues should be consulted prior to employing the technique. It is frustrating to find that an adequate deep cervical plexus block does not work for performance of carotid endarterectomy because of differing surgical expectations.

24

Stellate Block

Perspective

The primary use of stellate block is in diagnosis and treatment of sympathetic dystrophies of the upper extremity. It may also be used in clinical situations when increased perfusion to the upper extremity is desired, although this can also be accomplished by brachial plexus blockade.

Patient Selection. Patients for this block are primarily those with reflex sympathetic dystrophies of the upper extremity or those with impaired perfusion to the upper extremity following trauma.

Pharmacologic Choice. Even during diagnostic use of stellate ganglion block, it is often desirable to produce a long-lasting block. Therefore, a solution of 0.25% bupivacaine with 1:200,000 epinephrine is often my first choice.

Placement

Anatomy. The cervical sympathetic trunk is a cephalad continuation of the thoracic sympathetic trunk. It is composed of three ganglia: the superior cervical ganglion, generally opposite the first cervical vertebra; the middle cervical ganglion, usually opposite the sixth cervical vertebra; and the stellate (cervicothoracic ganglion), generally opposite the seventh cervical and first thoracic vertebrae. The stellate ganglion is a fusion of the lower cervical ganglion and the first thoracic ganglion—thus, the name cervicothoracic ganglion (Fig. 24–1). The cervical part of the sympathetic chain and ganglion lies on the anterior surface of, and is separated from, the transverse processes of the cervical vertebrae by the thin prevertebral musculature (primarily the longus colli muscle), as illustrated in Figure 24–2. Since the anterior approach to the stellate ganglion is often made at the level of the sixth cervical vertebral tubercle (Chassaignac's), it can be seen that the term *stellate block* is really a misnomer. To produce stellate (cervicothoracic) ganglion block, anesthesiologists must rely on spread of local anesthetic solution along the prevertebral muscles.

Position. The patient should be in the supine position, with the neck in slight extension (Fig. 24–3). This is often facilitated by removing the patient's pillow prior to positioning. The anesthesiologist should stand alongside the patient's neck, and the sixth cervical vertebral tubercle should be identified with palpation. This can be accomplished by locating the cricoid cartilage and moving the fingers laterally until they contact this easily palpable vertebral tubercle.

Needle Puncture. Once the sixth cervical vertebral tubercle is identified as shown in Figure 24–3, the anesthesiologist should

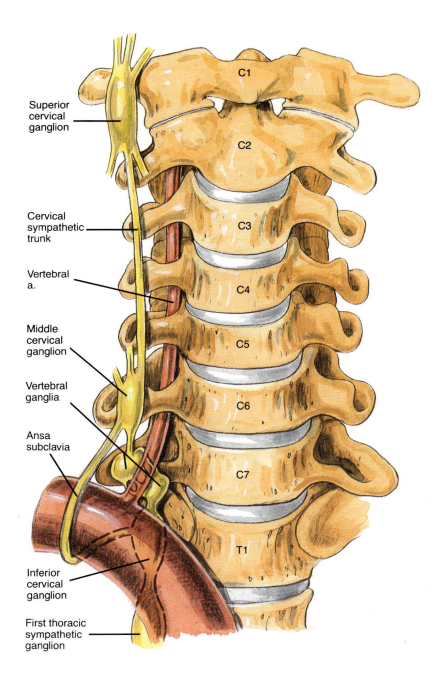

Figure 24–1 Stellate ganglion block—simplified sympathetic chain anatomy

Superior cervical ganglion

Cervical sympathetic trunk

Vertebral a.

Middle cervical ganglion

Vertebral ganglia

Ansa subclavia

Inferior cervical ganglion

First thoracic sympathetic ganglion

C1

C2

C3

C4

C5

C6

C7

T1

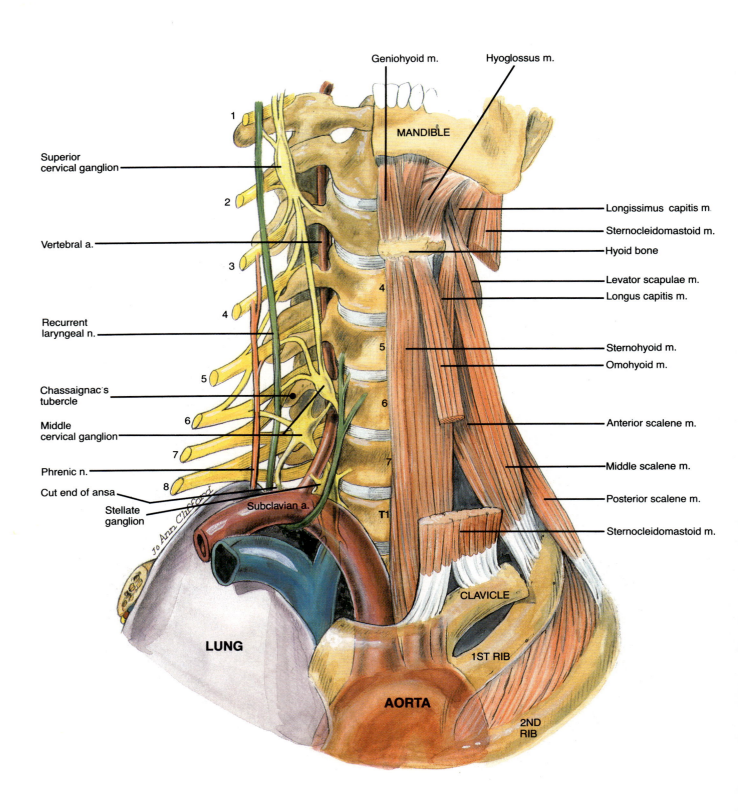

Geniohyoid m.

Hyoglossus m.

MANDIBLE

Superior
cervical ganglion

1

2

Longissimus capitis m.

Sternocleidomastoid m.

Vertebral a.

Hyoid bone

3

Levator scapulae m.

Longus capitis m.

4

Recurrent
laryngeal n.

5

Sternohyoid m.

Omohyoid m.

Chassaignac's
tubercle

5

6

Middle
cervical ganglion

6

Anterior scalene m.

7

Phrenic n.

7

Middle scalene m.

Cut end of ansa

8

Posterior scalene m.

Stellate
ganglion

Subclavian a.

Sternocleidomastoid m.

Jo Ann Clifford

T1

LUNG

CLAVICLE

1ST RIB

AORTA

2ND
RIB

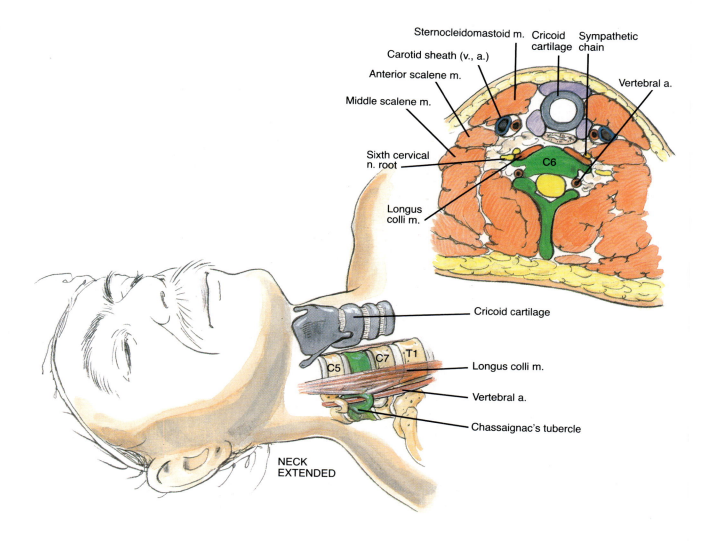

Sternocleidomastoid m.   Cricoid cartilage   Sympathetic chain

Carotid sheath (v., a.)

Anterior scalene m.

Middle scalene m.

Vertebral a.

Sixth cervical n. root

C6

Longus colli m.

Cricoid cartilage

C5   C7   T1

Longus colli m.

Vertebral a.

Chassaignac's tubercle

NECK EXTENDED

place the index and third fingers between the carotid artery laterally and the trachea medially at the level of C6. A short, 22- or 25-gauge needle is then inserted until it contacts the transverse process of C6. The needle is then withdrawn approximately 1 to 2 mm, and injection of 5 to 10 ml of local anesthetic is carried out (Fig. 24–4).

Potential Problems. As illustrated in Figure 24–2, the vertebral artery runs in close proximity to the transverse process of C6, and intravascular injection must be guarded against. The recurrent laryngeal and phrenic nerves may also be blocked if needle position is not ideal. Patients should be cautioned that they may experience a lump in their throat

or a sense of dyspnea. Reassurance is usually all that is necessary.

Pearls

The most useful maneuver to facilitate this block is to use the index and third finger of the palpating hand to compress the tissues overlying the sixth cervical vertebral tubercle. The patient will experience some deep pressure discomfort from this maneuver, but clear identification of the tubercle will make this block efficient, and most patients are willing to accept the deep discomfort if the block is carried out efficiently.

Figure 24–3 Stellate block anatomy—surface and cross-sectional

Figure 24–4 Stellate block—anatomy and technique

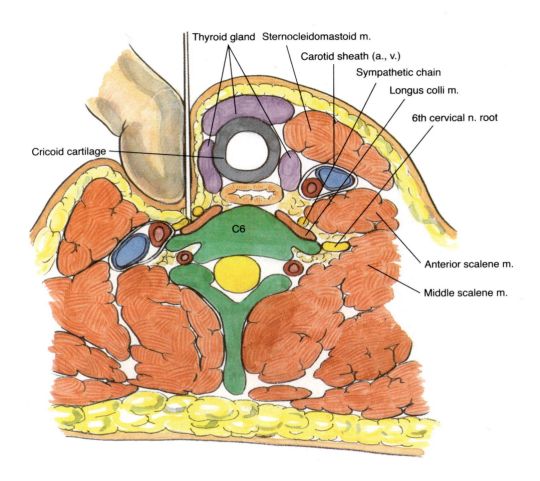

Thyroid gland Sternocleidomastoid m.

Carotid sheath (a., v.)

Sympathetic chain

Longus colli m.

6th cervical n. root

Cricoid cartilage

C6

Anterior scalene m.

Middle scalene m.

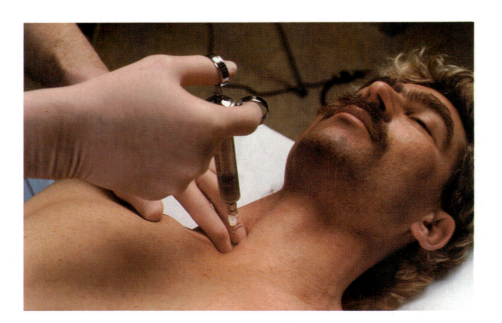

25

Airway Block Anatomy

If there is one regional block that an anesthesiologist should master, it is airway blockade. Even those anesthesiologist who prefer to use general anesthesia for the majority of their cases will be faced with the necessity of providing airway blockade prior to anesthetic induction in patients who may have airway compromise, trauma to the upper airway, or unstable cervical vertebrae. As illustrated in Figure 25–1, innervation of the airway can be separated into three principal neural pathways. If nasal intubation is planned, some method of anesthetizing maxillary branches from the trigeminal nerve will need to be carried out. As our manipulations involve the pharynx and posterior third of the tongue, glossopharyngeal block will be required. Structures more distal in the airway to the epiglottis will require blockade of vagal branches.

Specific glossopharyngeal nerves that are of interest to anesthesiologists who undertake airway anesthesia are the pharyngeal nerves, which are primarily sensory to the pharyngeal mucosa; the tonsillar nerves, which provide sensation to the mucosa overlying the palatine tonsil and contiguous parts of the soft palate; and sensory branches to the posterior one third of the tongue. The glossopharyngeal nerve exits from the skull via the jugular foramen in close contact with the spinal accessory nerve. As the glossopharyngeal exits from the jugular foramen, it is also in close contact with the vagus nerve that likewise travels within the carotid sheath in the upper portion of the neck.

The vagus nerve supplies innervation to the mucosa of the airway from the level of the epiglottis to the distal airways, through both the superior and recurrent laryngeal nerves, as illustrated in Figures 25–2 and 25–3. Although the vagus is primarily a parasympathetic nerve, it also contains some fibers from the cervical sympathetic chain, as well as motor fibers to laryngeal muscles. The superior laryngeal nerve provides sensation to both sides of the epiglottis and airway mucosa to the level of the vocal cords. It provides innervation to the mucosa after entering the thyrohyoid membrane just inferior to the hyoid bone between the greater and lesser cornua of the hyoid. This mucosal innervation is carried out through the internal laryngeal nerve, a branch of the superior laryngeal nerve. The superior laryngeal nerve also continues as the external laryngeal nerve along the exterior of the larynx; it provides motor innervation to the cricothyroid muscle.

The recurrent laryngeal nerve is a branch of the vagus that ascends along the posterior

Figure 25–1 Airway blocks—simplified functional anatomy

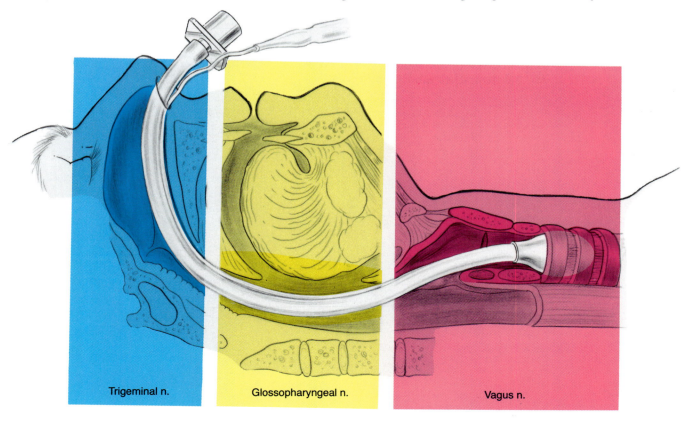

| Trigeminal n. | Glossopharyngeal n. | Vagus n. |

Figure 25—2 Airway block anatomy—laryngeal innervation

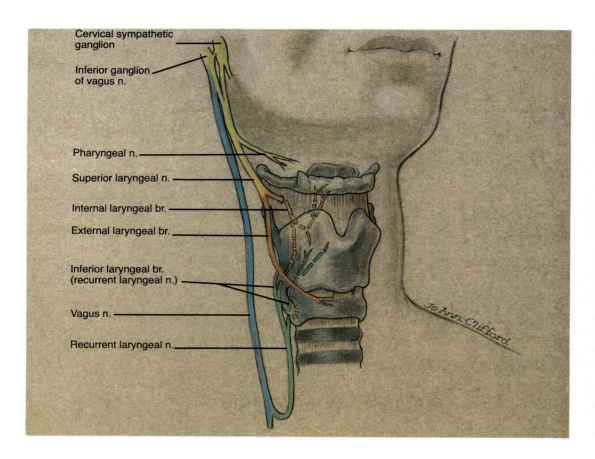

Cervical sympathetic ganglion

Inferior ganglion of vagus n.

Pharyngeal n.

Superior laryngeal n.

Internal laryngeal br.

External laryngeal br.

Inferior laryngeal br. (recurrent laryngeal n.)

Vagus n.

Recurrent laryngeal n.

Jo Ann Clifford

lateral margin of the trachea after looping under the right subclavian artery as it leaves the vagus nerve on the right or around the left side of the arch of the aorta, lateral to the ligamentum arteriosum on the left. The recurrent nerves ascend and innervate the larynx and the trachea caudal to the vocal cords. This anatomy is illustrated in Figures 25—2, 25—3, and 25—4. Figure 25—5 demonstrates a sagittal magnetic resonance image with an interpretive illustration of airway innervation keyed to colors used in Figure 25—1.

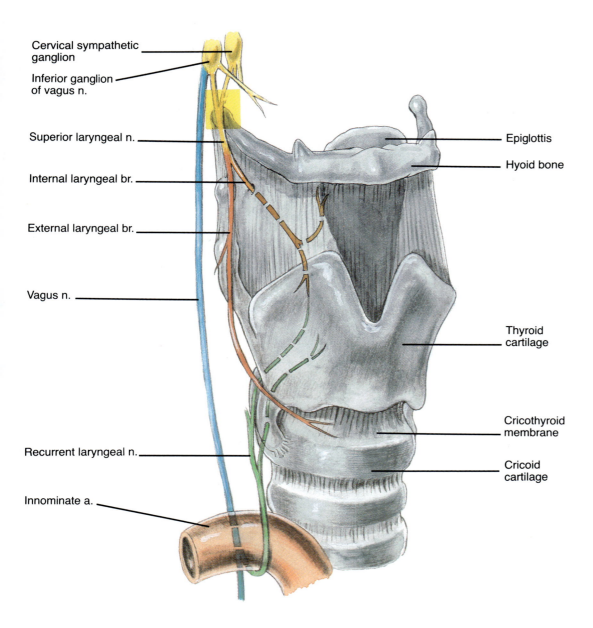

Cervical sympathetic
ganglion

Inferior ganglion
of vagus n.

Superior laryngeal n.

Internal laryngeal br.

External laryngeal br.

Vagus n.

Recurrent laryngeal n.

Innominate a.

Epiglottis

Hyoid bone

Thyroid
cartilage

Cricothyroid
membrane

Cricoid
cartilage

Figure 25–3 Airway block anatomy—laryngeal vagal and sympathetic connection

Figure 25–4 Airway block anatomy— laryngeal structures and simplified innervation

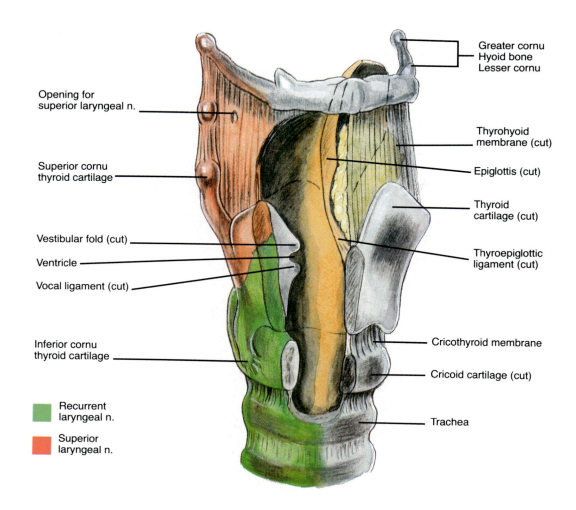

Opening for superior laryngeal n.

Superior cornu thyroid cartilage

Vestibular fold (cut)

Ventricle

Vocal ligament (cut)

Inferior cornu thyroid cartilage

Greater cornu
Hyoid bone
Lesser cornu

Thyrohyoid membrane (cut)

Epiglottis (cut)

Thyroid cartilage (cut)

Thyroepiglottic ligament (cut)

Cricothyroid membrane

Cricoid cartilage (cut)

Trachea

Recurrent laryngeal n.

Superior laryngeal n.

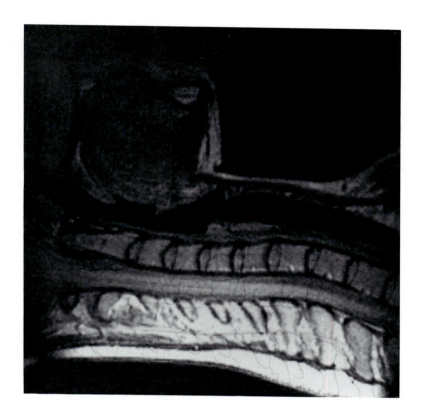

Figure 25–5 Airway block sagittal anatomy—magnetic resonance section and interpretive line drawing

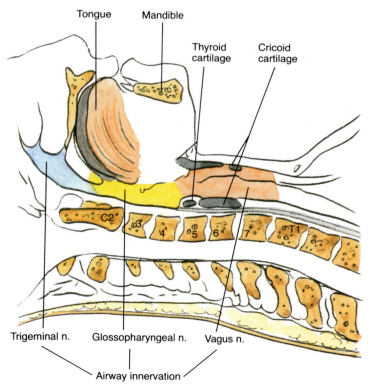

26

Glossopharyngeal Block

Perspective

Glossopharyngeal block is useful for anesthesia of the mucosa of the pharynx and soft palate, as well as eliminating the gag reflex that results when pressure is applied to the posterior one third of the tongue.

Patient Selection. Glossopharyngeal block can be used in most patients needing atraumatic, sedated, spontaneously ventilating, "awake" tracheal intubation.

Pharmacologic Choice. The local anesthetic chosen for glossopharyngeal block does not need to provide motor blockade. Lidocaine (0.5%) is an appropriate choice of local anesthetic.

Placement

Anatomy. The glossopharyngeal nerve exits from the jugular foramina at the base of the skull, as illustrated in Figure 26−1, in

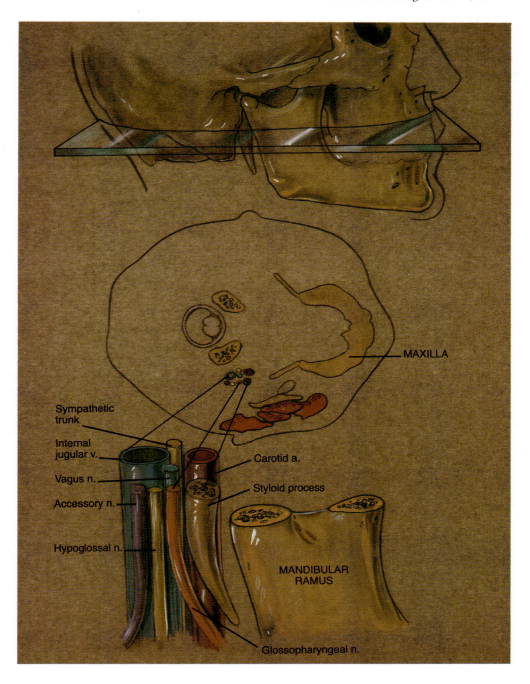

Figure 26−1 Glossopharyngeal block—peristyloid anatomy—cross-sectional view with detail

MAXILLA

Sympathetic trunk

Internal jugular v.

Vagus n.

Accessory n.

Hypoglossal n.

Carotid a.

Styloid process

MANDIBULAR RAMUS

Glossopharyngeal n.

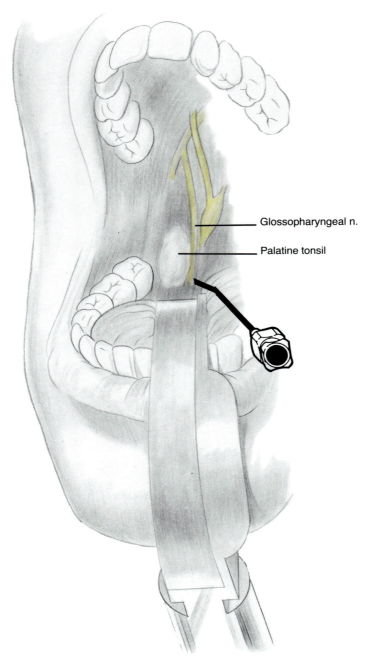

Glossopharyngeal n.

Palatine tonsil

Figure 26–2 Glossopharyngeal block—intraoral anatomy and technique

close association with other structures of the carotid sheath, vagus nerve, and styloid process. The glossopharyngeal nerve descends in the neck, passes between the internal carotid and external carotid arteries on its way to dividing into pharyngeal branches and motor branches to the stylopharyngeus muscle, as well as branches innervating the area of the palatine tonsil and the posterior third of the tongue. These distal branches of the glossopharyngeal nerve are located submucosally immediately posterior to the palatine tonsil, deep to the posterior tonsillar pillar.

Position. Glossopharyngeal block can be carried out intraorally or in a peristyloid manner. If the block is to be carried out intraorally, the patient must be able to open the mouth, and sufficient topical anesthesia of the tongue must be provided to allow needle placement at the base of the posterior tonsillar pillar. If the block is to be carried out in a peristyloid manner, the patient does not need to have the capability of opening the mouth.

Needle Puncture—Intraoral Glossopharyngeal Block. Following topical anesthesia of the tongue, the patient's mouth is opened widely and the posterior tonsillar pillar (palatopharyngeal fold) is identified by using a no. 3 Macintosh laryngoscope blade. Then, an angled, 22-gauge, 9-cm needle (see comment in Pearls section) is inserted at the caudad portion of the posterior tonsillar pillar. The needle tip is inserted submucosally, and, following careful aspiration for blood, 5 ml of local anesthetic is injected. The block is then repeated on the contralateral side (Fig. 26–2).

Needle Puncture—Peristyloid Approach. The patient lies in a supine position, with the head in a neutral position. Marks are placed on the mastoid process and the angle of the mandible, as illustrated in Figure 26–3. A line is drawn between these two marks, and at the midpoint of that line the needle is inserted to contact the styloid process. To facilitate styloid identification, a finger palpates the styloid process with deep pressure and, although this can be uncomfortable for the patient, the short 22-gauge needle is then inserted until it impinges upon the styloid pro-

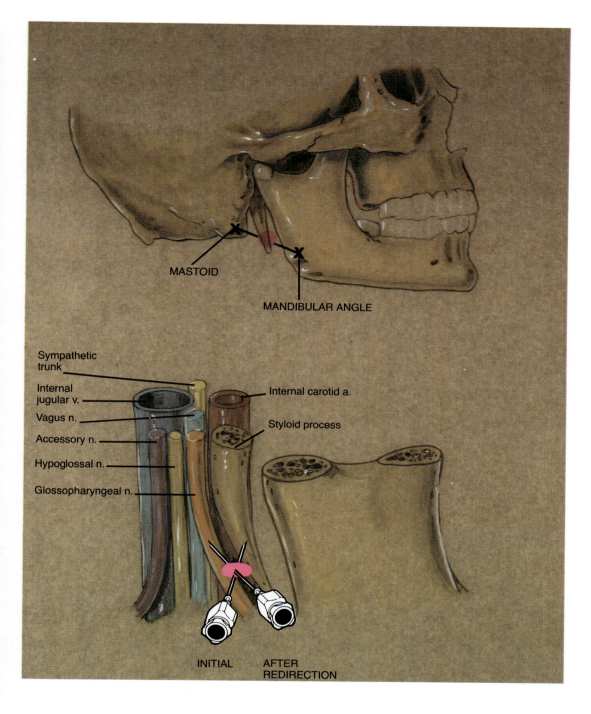

MASTOID

MANDIBULAR ANGLE

Sympathetic trunk

Internal jugular v.

Vagus n.

Accessory n.

Hypoglossal n.

Glossopharyngeal n.

Internal carotid a.

Styloid process

INITIAL   AFTER REDIRECTION

Figure 26–3 Glossopharyngeal block—peristyloid technique

cess. This needle is then withdrawn and redirected off the styloid process posteriorly. As soon as bony contact is lost and there is negative aspiration for blood, 5 to 7 ml of local anesthetic is injected. The block can then be repeated on the contralateral side.

Potential Problems. Both the intraoral and peristyloid blocks have few complications if careful aspiration for blood is carried out during the technique. In the peristyloid approach, the glossopharyngeal nerve is closely related to both the internal jugular vein and internal carotid artery. In the intraoral approach, the terminal branches of the glossopharyngeal nerves are closely related to the internal carotid arteries, which lie immediately lateral to the needle tips if they are correctly positioned.

Pearls

A frequent problem with the intraoral glossopharyngeal block is finding a needle to use for blockade. This problem can be easily overcome by using a 22-gauge disposable spinal needle. In an aseptic manner the stylet should be removed from the disposable spinal needle and discarded. Subsequently utilizing the sterile container that the 22-gauge spinal needle was packaged in, the distal 1 cm of the needle is bent to allow more controlled submucosal insertion.

When airway anesthesia for sedated, spontaneously ventilating, "awake" tracheal intubation is necessary, this block should be utilized more frequently than it is. I believe that the block is effective in further reducing the gag reflex that results from pressure on the posterior one third of the tongue, even after adequate topical mucosal anesthesia has been obtained.

27

Superior Laryngeal Block

Perspective

The superior laryngeal nerve block is useful as one of the methods of providing airway anesthesia. Block of the superior laryngeal nerve can provide anesthesia of the larynx from the epiglottis to the level of the vocal cords.

Patient Selection. This block may be appropriate for any patient requiring tracheal intubation prior to anesthetic induction.

Pharmacologic Choice. Lidocaine (0.5%) is an appropriate local anesthetic for this block.

Placement

Anatomy. The superior laryngeal nerve is a branch of the vagus nerve. After it leaves the main vagal trunk, it courses through the neck and passes medially, caudal to the greater cornu of the hyoid bone, at which point it divides into an internal branch and an external branch. The internal branch is the nerve of interest in superior laryngeal nerve block, and it is blocked where it enters the thyrohyoid membrane just inferior to the caudal aspect of the hyoid bone (Fig. 27–1).

Position. The patient is placed supine, with the neck extended. The anesthesiologist should displace the hyoid bone toward the side to be blocked by grasping the hyoid between the index finger and thumb (Fig. 27–2). A 25-gauge, short needle is then inserted to make contact with the greater cornu of the hyoid. The needle is walked off the caudal edge of the hyoid and advanced 2 to 3 mm so that the needle tip rests between the thyrohyoid membrane laterally and the laryngeal mucosa medially. Two to three milliliters of the drug is then injected; an additional 1 ml is injected while withdrawing the needle.

Potential Problems. It is possible to place the needle into the interior of the larynx with this approach, although that should not result in long-term problems. If the block is carried out as described, intravascular injection should be infrequent, in spite of the superior laryngeal artery and vein piercing the thyrohyoid membrane with the internal laryngeal nerve.

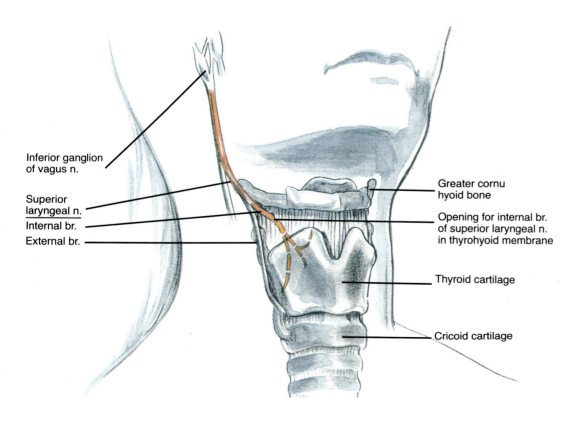

Figure 27–1 Superior laryngeal nerve block—anatomy

Inferior ganglion of vagus n.

Superior laryngeal n.
Internal br.
External br.

Greater cornu hyoid bone

Opening for internal br. of superior laryngeal n. in thyrohyoid membrane

Thyroid cartilage

Cricoid cartilage

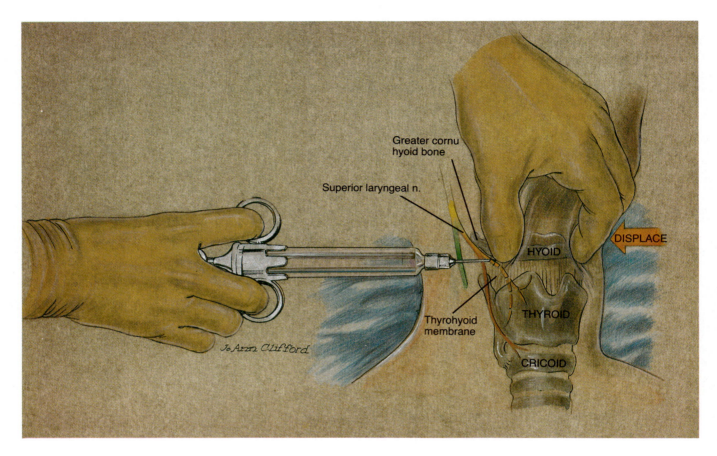

Figure 27–2 Superior laryngeal nerve block—technique

Pearls

One help when performing this block is to firmly displace the hyoid bone toward the side to be blocked, even if it causes the patient some minor discomfort. The dis-comfort usually can be minimized by appropriate amounts of sedation. If a 3-ring syringe is utilized, the sedation, coupled with an efficient block, provides an acceptable block for both patient and anesthesiologist.

28

Translaryngeal Block

Perspective

This block, as all airway blocks, can be useful during sedated, spontaneously ventilating, "awake" tracheal intubation.

Patient Selection. Any patient is a candidate in whom it is desirable to avoid the Valsalva-like straining that may follow "awake" (sedated and spontaneously ventilating) tracheal intubation.

Pharmacologic Choice. The local anesthetic most often chosen for this block is 3 to 4 ml of 4% lidocaine. When multiple airway blocks are administered, the total dose of local anesthetic used should be kept in mind.

Placement

Anatomy. Translaryngeal block is most useful in providing topical anesthesia to the laryngotracheal mucosa innervated by branches of the vagus nerve. Both surfaces of the epiglottis and laryngeal structures to the level of the vocal cords receive innervation through the internal branch of the superior laryngeal nerve, a branch of the vagus. Distal airway mucosa also receives innervation through the vagus nerve but via the recurrent laryngeal nerve. Translaryngeal injection of local anesthetic is helpful in providing topical anesthesia for both these vagal branches, since injection below the cords through the cricothyroid membrane results in solution being spread onto tracheal structures, as well as being coughed onto more superior laryngeal structures (Fig. 28–1).

Position. The patient should be in a supine position, with the pillow removed and the neck slightly extended. As illustrated in Figure 28–2, the anesthetist should be in position to place the index and third fingers in

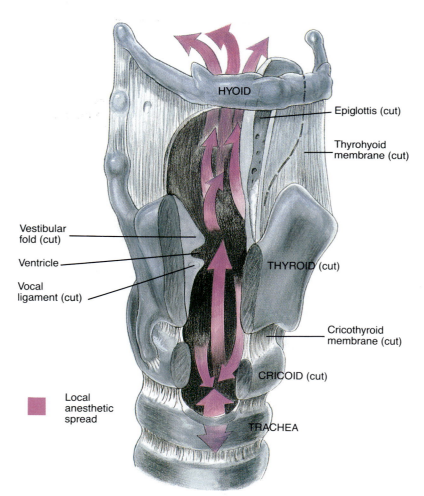

Figure 28–1 Translaryngeal block—anatomy and local anesthetic spread

HYOID

Epiglottis (cut)

Thyrohyoid membrane (cut)

Vestibular fold (cut)

Ventricle

Vocal ligament (cut)

THYROID (cut)

Cricothyroid membrane (cut)

CRICOID (cut)

Local anesthetic spread

TRACHEA

Figure 28–2 Translaryngeal block—anatomy and technique

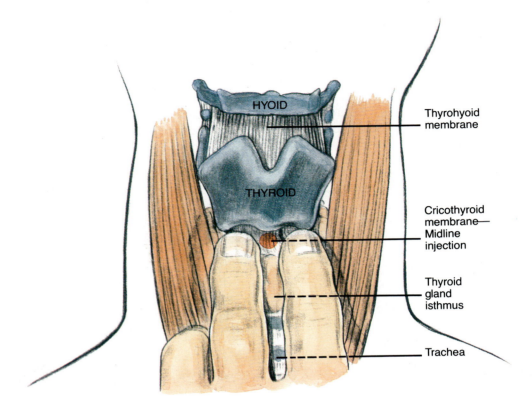

HYOID

THYROID

Thyrohyoid membrane

Cricothyroid membrane— Midline injection

Thyroid gland isthmus

Trachea

the space between the thyroid and cricoid cartilages (cricothyroid membrane).

Needle Puncture. The cricothyroid membrane should be localized, the midline identified, and the needle, 22-gauge or smaller, inserted into the midline until air can be freely aspirated. When air can be freely aspirated, the 3 ml of local anesthetic is rapidly injected. The needle should be removed immediately, since it is almost inevitable that patients cough at this point. Conversely, a needle-over-the-catheter assembly (IV catheter) can be used for the block. Once air is aspirated, the inner needle is removed and the injection performed through the catheter.

Potential Problems. This block can result in coughing, which should be considered in patients in whom coughing is clearly undesirable. The midline should be used for needle insertion, since the area is nearly devoid of major vascular structures. Conversely, the needle does not need to be misplaced far off the midline to encounter significant arterial and venous vessels.

Pearls

This block is most effectively utilized after the patient has been appropriately sedated. There has long been a belief that this block should be used cautiously, if at all, in patients at high risk for gastric aspiration. My own belief is that the block is more frequently misused by not being applied in appropriate situations than by being applied when the patient is at risk for gastric aspiration.

Another hint is to perform the local anesthetic injection after asking the patient to forcefully exhale. This forces the patient to initially inspire prior to coughing, making distal airway anesthesia predictable.

29

Truncal Anatomy

A number of regional anesthetic techniques rely on blockade of the thoracic or lumbar somatic nerves. As illustrated in Figure 29–1, thoracic and lumbar somatic innervation extends from the chest and axilla to the toes. Although few major surgical procedures can be carried out during somatic blockade alone, appropriate use of somatic block with long-acting local anesthetics provides unique and useful analgesia. Also, when even longer-acting local anesthetics become available, possibly some form of thoracic or lumbar somatic nerve block, such as intercostal nerve block, will be able to provide even more useful postoperative analgesia.

Figure 29–1 Truncal anatomy—dermatomes

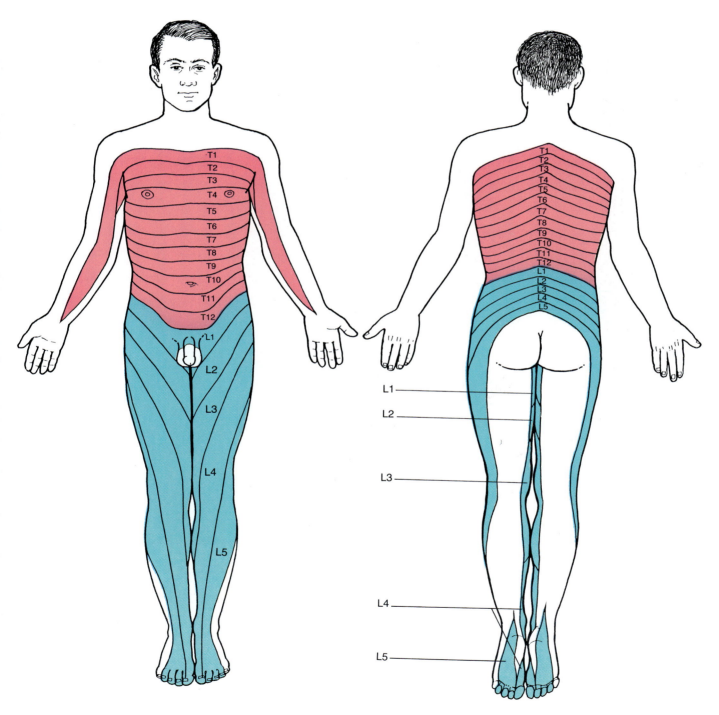

One of the advantages that somatic blockade has over centroneuraxis blocks is the ability to avoid widespread interruption of the sympathetic nervous system with the somatic blocks. As shown in Figure 29–2, the major somatic nerves are the ventral rami of the thoracic and lumbar nerves. Additionally, as shown in the inset in Figure 29–2, the nerves contribute preganglionic sympathetic fibers to the sympathetic chain through the white rami communicantes and receive postganglionic neurons from the sympathetic chain through gray rami communicantes. These rami from the sympathetic system connect to the spinal nerves near their exit from the intervertebral foramina. The dorsal rami of these spinal nerves provide innervation to dorsal midline structures.

Figure 29–2 Truncal anatomy—cross-sectional view

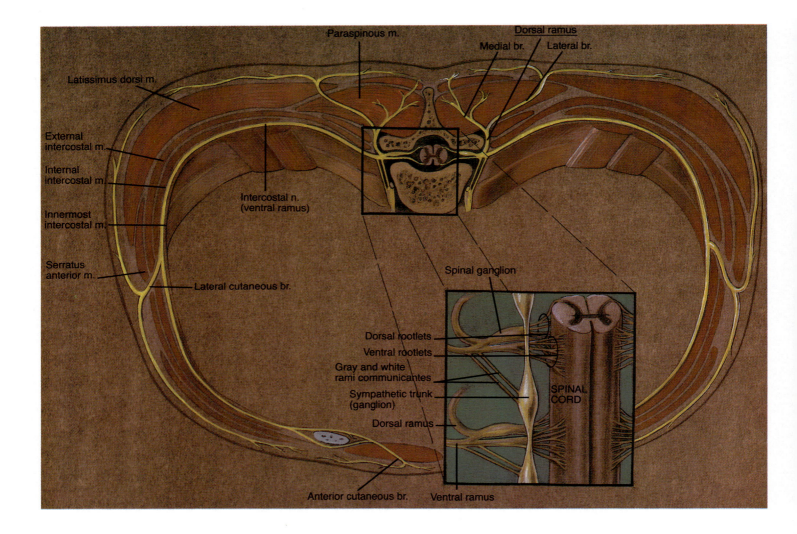

30

Breast Block

Perspective

There is increasing emphasis on carrying out ''lesser'' surgical procedures for breast cancer. These lesser procedures often involve lumpectomy or simple mastectomy and avoid extensive chest wall procedures that in the past also involved shoulder structures. For this reason, breast blocks may become more appropriate for women undergoing operation for breast cancer.

Patient Selection. Any individuals requiring breast surgical procedures are candidates for breast block, although appropriate sedation for the block and procedure must be constantly kept in mind.

Pharmacologic Choice. This block is designed to provide sensory block rather than motor blockade. For that reason, lower concentrations of local anesthetic are possible. For example, 0.75% to 1% lidocaine or mepivacaine are possibilities, and 0.25% bupivacaine is also appropriate.

Placement

Anatomy. The nerves that must be blocked to carry out the breast block are the second through seventh intercostal nerves and some terminal branches from the superficial cervical plexus (Fig. 30–1).

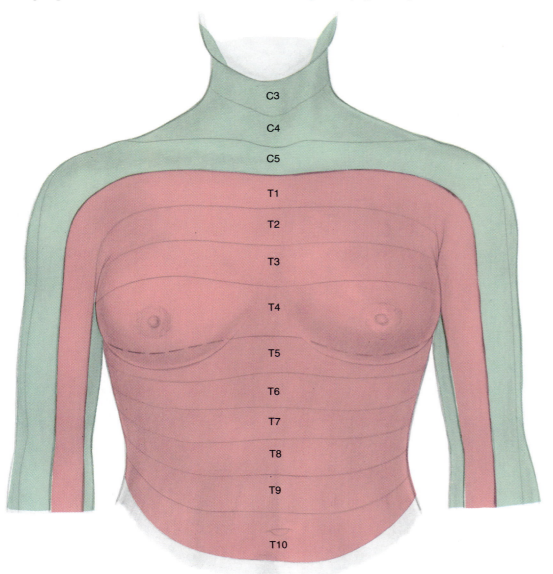

Figure 30–1 Breast block anatomy—dermatomes

Position. This block can be carried out with the patient in the supine position, if blockade of the intercostal nerves is undertaken in the midaxillary line. Conversely, these same nerves can be blocked from a posterior approach if the patient is placed in the prone position.

Needle Puncture. This block can be carried out with the patient in the supine position by performing intercostal nerve block from T2 to T7 in the patient's midaxillary line, as shown in Figure 30–2A. The patient's arm should be abducted at the shoulder and placed on an arm board, or "tucked under" the head as shown in Figure 30–2A. The intercostal nerve block can be carried out by utilizing a 22-gauge, short-beveled, 3-cm needle and placing 5 ml of local anesthetic solution inferior to each rib, after walking the needle tip off each rib's inferior border. If insufficient

Figure 30–2 Breast block—positioning and technique

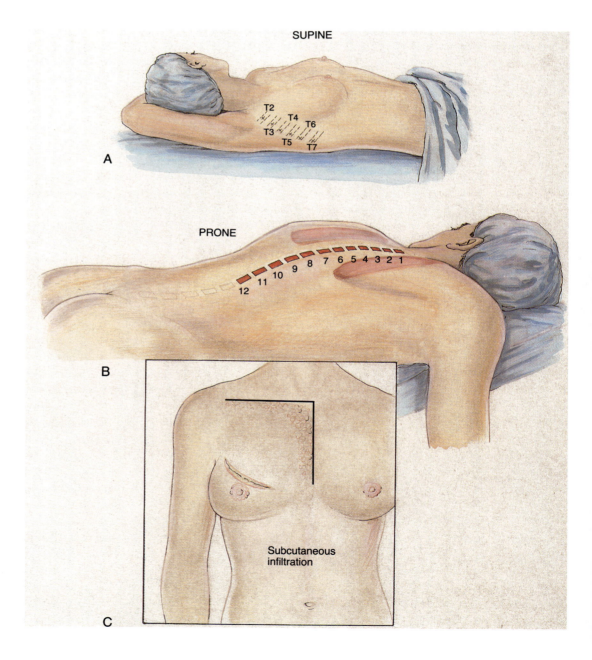

analgesia is produced, subcutaneous infiltration may need to be added, since the lateral cutaneous branches of the intercostal nerve may have been missed. This is possible since the lateral cutaneous nerve may branch more posteriorly in some patients. In addition to the intercostal nerve block, subcutaneous infiltration of local anesthetic needs to be performed in an "upside-down L" pattern, as shown in Figure 30–2C. This infraclavicular infiltration needs to be added to interrupt those branches of the superficial cervical plexus that provide sensation to portions of the upper chest wall. Additionally, subcutaneous infiltration in the midline is required to block those intercostal nerve fibers that cross the midline from the contralateral side. The subcutaneous infiltration is facilitated if a 10- to 12-cm needle is used.

If a posterior approach to the intercostal nerves is utilized, the patient must be placed in the prone position and intercostal nerve block carried out by walking the needle off, and immediately inferior to, the rib from T2 through T7 (Fig. 30–2B). The technique is detailed in Chapter 31, Intercostal Nerve Block. If the posterior approach is chosen, the subcutaneous infiltration, as previously outlined, must also be added.

Potential Problems. Pneumothorax can occur with this technique, although it should be infrequent.

Pearls

Owing to the understandable anxiety that often accompanies breast surgery, patients should understand prior to undertaking this anesthetic approach that heavy sedation is most often appropriate in combination with the breast block. Likewise, in some patients, the maintenance of a "sense of control" during reconstructive or augmentation breast operation makes them ideal candidates for a technique in which a loss of control accompanying general anesthesia is avoided.

31

Intercostal Block

Perspective

Intercostal nerve blocks provide unexcelled analgesia of the body wall. Thus, it is appropriate to use the technique for analgesia following upper abdominal and thoracic surgery or for rib fracture analgesia. It is possible to perform minor surgical procedures on the chest or abdominal wall using only intercostal blocks, but, in general, some supplementation is most often appropriate to complement this block. This block can also be used when chest tubes (thoracostomy tubes) are placed or when feeding gastrostomy tubes are inserted.

Patient Selection. All patients are candidates for this block, though it should be realized that as patients become more obese the blocks are technically more difficult to carry out.

Pharmacologic Choice. Like any decision about local anesthetic choice, it must be decided whether motor blockade will be required for a successful block. If intercostal nerve block is combined with light general anesthesia for intra-abdominal surgery and the intercostal block is wanted to provide abdominal muscle relaxation, a higher concentration of local anesthetic will be needed. In this setting, 0.5% bupivacaine, 1.5% lidocaine, or 1.5% mepivacaine is an appropriate choice. Conversely, if sensory analgesia is all that is necessary from the block, then 0.25% bupivacaine, 1% lidocaine, or 1% mepivacaine is appropriate.

Placement

Anatomy. Intercostal nerves are the ventral rami of T1 through T11. The 12th thoracic nerve travels a subcostal course and is technically not an intercostal nerve. The subcostal nerve can provide branches to the ilioinguinal and iliohypogastric nerves. Some fibers from the first thoracic nerve also unite with fibers from C8 to form the lowest trunk of the brachial plexus. The other notable variation in intercostal nerve anatomy is the contribution of some fibers from T2 and T3 to the formation of the intercostobrachial nerve. The terminal distribution of this nerve is to the skin of the medial aspect of the upper arm.

Examination of an individual intercostal nerve shows that there are five principal branches (Fig. 31–1). The intercostal nerve contributes preganglionic sympathetic fibers to the sympathetic chain through the white rami communicantes *(branch 1)* and receives postganglionic neurons from the sympathetic chain ganglion through the gray rami communicantes *(branch 2)*. These rami are joined to the spinal nerves near their exit from the intervertebral foramina. Also, shortly following exit from the intervertebral foramina, the dorsal rami carrying posterior cutaneous and motor fibers *(branch 3)* supply skin and muscles in the paravertebral region. The lateral cutaneous branch of the intercostal nerve arises just anterior to the midaxillary line before sending subcutaneous fibers posteriorly and anteriorly *(branch 4)*. The termination of the intercostal nerve is known as the anterior cutaneous branch *(branch 5)*. Medial to the angle of the rib, the intercostal nerve lies between the pleura and the internal intercostal fascia. In the paravertebral region, there is only loose areolar and fatty tissue between the nerve and pleura. At the rib's posterior angle, the area most commonly used during intercostal nerve block, the nerve lies between the internal intercostal muscles and the intercostalis intimus muscle. Throughout the intercostal nerve course, the nerve traverses the intercostal spaces inferior to the intercostal artery and vein of the same space.

Position. To block the intercostal nerve in its preferred location—that is, just lateral to the paraspinous muscles at the angle of the ribs—the patient ideally is placed in the prone position. A pillow should be placed under the patient's midabdomen to reduce the lumbar lordosis and to accentuate the intercostal spaces posteriorly. The arms should be allowed to hang down from the edge of the block table (or gurney) to allow the scapula to rotate as far laterally as possible.

Needle Puncture. It is advisable to use a marking pen to outline pertinent anatomy for most regional blocks, and in no block is this more important than in the intercostal nerve block. The midline should be marked from T1 to L5, then two paramedian lines should be drawn at the posterior angle of the ribs. These lines should angle medially in the upper thoracic region, so as to parallel the medial edge of the scapula. By successfully

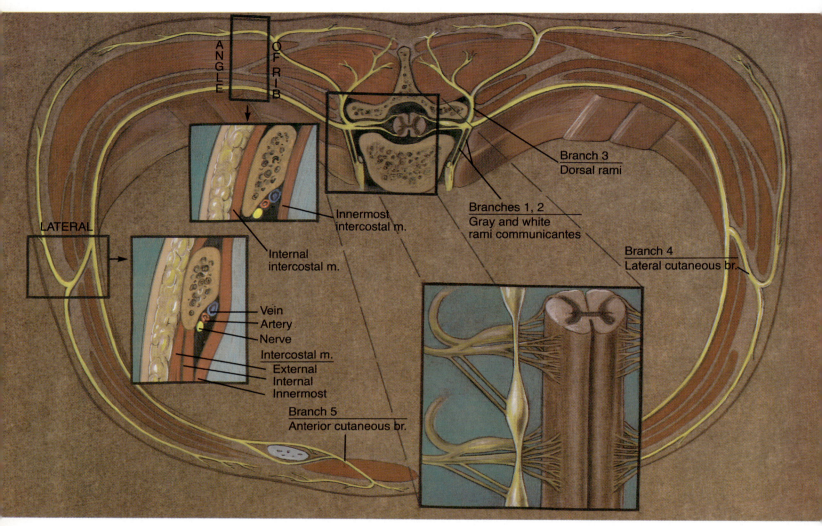

ANGLE
OF RIB

LATERAL

Innermost
intercostal m.

Internal
intercostal m.

Vein
Artery
Nerve
Intercostal m.
External
Internal
Innermost

Branch 5
Anterior cutaneous br.

Branch 3
Dorsal rami

Branches 1, 2
Gray and white
rami communicantes

Branch 4
Lateral cutaneous br.

Figure 31–1 Intercostal nerve block—cross-sectional anatomy

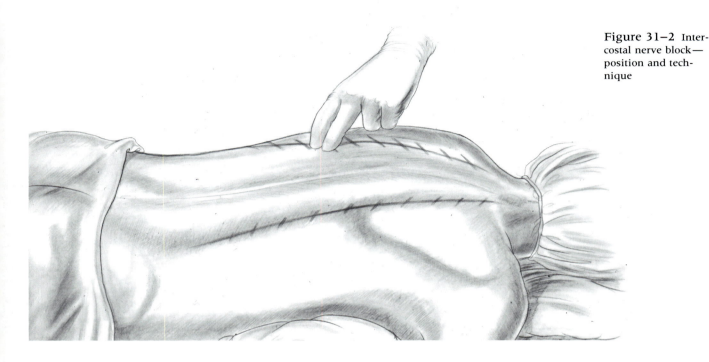

Figure 31—2 Intercostal nerve block— position and technique

palpating and marking the inferior edge of each rib along these two paramedian lines, a diagram like that in Figure 31—2 is created. Prior to needle puncture, appropriate intravenous sedation should be administered to produce amnesia and analgesia during the multiple injections needed for the block. Barbiturates, benzodiazepines, ketamine, or short-acting opioids can be combined. Skin wheals are raised with a 30-gauge needle at each of the previously marked sites of injection, and then intercostal block is carried out bilaterally. As illustrated in Figure 31—3, a 22-gauge, short-beveled, 3- to 4-cm needle is attached to a 10-ml control syringe. It is important that the hand and finger positions illustrated in Figure 31—3 are adhered to and incorporated into the development of each anesthesiologist's own systematic technique.

Beginning at the most caudal rib to be blocked, the index and third fingers of the left hand are used to retract the skin up and over the rib. The needle should be introduced through the skin between the tips of the retracting fingers and advanced until it

contacts rib. It is important not to allow the needle to enter to a depth greater than the depth the palpating fingers define as rib. Once the needle contacts the rib, the right hand firmly maintains this contact while the left hand is shifted to hold the needle's hub and shaft between the thumb, index, and middle fingers. It is emphasized that the left hand's hypothenar eminence should be firmly placed against the patient's back. This hand placement allows maximal control of the needle depth as the left hand "walks" the needle off the inferior margin of the rib and into the intercostal groove—that is, a distance of 2 to 4 mm past the edge of the rib. With the needle in position, 3 to 5 ml of local anesthetic solution is injected. The process is then repeated for each of the nerves to be blocked. It is emphasized that in certain patients with cachexia or severe barrel chest deformity, the intercostal injection can be most effectively carried out with an even shorter 23- or 25-gauge needle.

Intercostal blockade at the posterior angle of the rib is not the only method applicable

Figure 31–3 Intercostal nerve block— stepwise technique 1–6

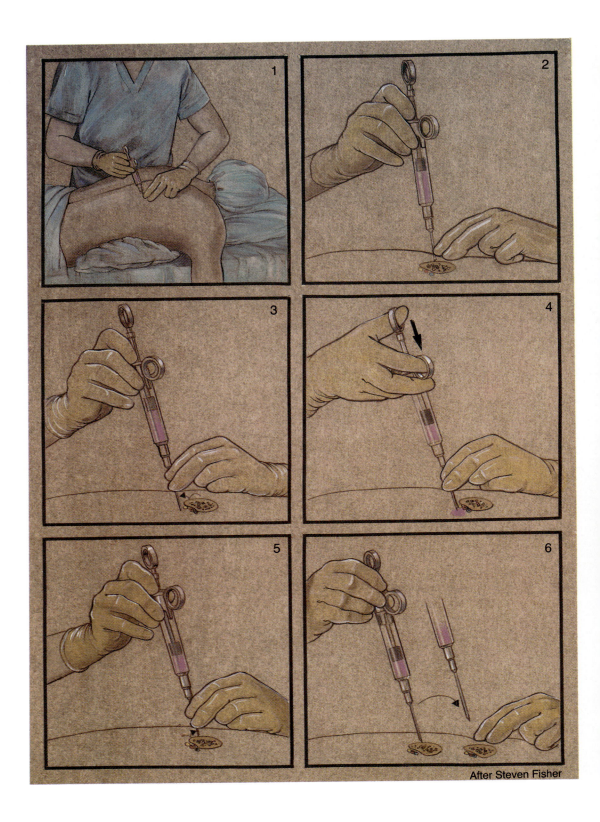

After Steven Fisher

to clinical regional anesthesia. As outlined in Chapter 30, Breast Block, intercostal block also can be effectively carried out at the mid-axillary line while the patient is in a supine position (Fig. 31–4). This position is clinically more convenient in many situations and probably under-utilized. One concern some raise with the lateral approach to the intercostal nerve is that the lateral cutaneous branch of the intercostal nerve might be missed with the approach. Clinically, this does not seem to be the case, and this observation is supported by computed tomographic studies showing that injected solutions spread readily along the subcostal groove for a distance of many centimeters. Therefore, even when lateral intercostal blockade is carried out, the lateral branch should be bathed with local anesthetic solution.

Potential Problems. The principal concern with intercostal nerve block is pneumothorax. Although the incidence of this complication is extremely low, many physicians avoid this block because of the imagined high frequency and seriousness of complications. Data suggest that the incidence of pneumothorax is less than half of 1%, and, even when it occurs, careful clinical observation is usually all that is necessary. The incidence of symptomatic pneumothorax following intercostal block is even lower—approximately 1:1000. If treatment is deemed necessary,

needle aspiration often can be carried out with successful re-expansion of the lung. Chest tube drainage should be performed only if there is a failure of lung re-expansion after observation or percutaneous aspiration.

As a result of the vascularity of the intercostal space, blood levels of local anesthetic are higher for multiple-level intercostal block than for any other standard regional anesthetic technique. Since these peak blood levels may be delayed for 15 to 20 minutes, patients should be closely monitored following the completion of a block for at least that interval.

Pearls

Effective intercostal nerve block requires adequate sedation. Patients are sedated so that they are able to lie comfortably on the table during the block. Combinations of sedatives seem to be the most effective, and, by combining a benzodiazepine, a short-acting narcotic, and/or ketamine, patients readily accept the procedure. Each anesthesiologist should develop a "recipe" for sedation since it is so important. Likewise, each anesthesiologist should develop a consistent method of hand and needle control for the block.

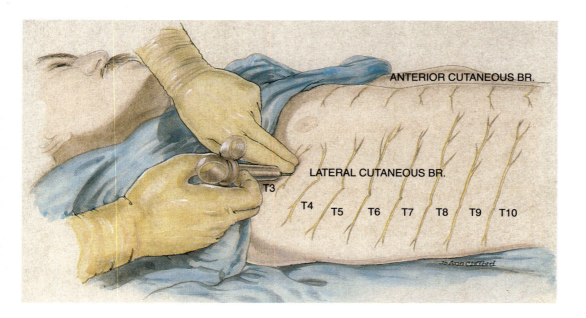

Figure 31–4 Intercostal nerve block—lateral technique

32

Interpleural Anesthesia

Perspective

Interpleural anesthesia is a technique that has developed in an attempt to "simplify" body wall and visceral anesthesia following upper abdominal or thoracic surgery. Although considerable research has been carried out on the technique, accurate stratification of the risk and benefit of interpleural anesthesia remains elusive.

Patient Selection. Patients undergoing upper abdominal or flank surgery or those recovering from fractured ribs have been the patients most frequently selected for interpleural anesthesia. Again, the appropriate selection of these patients remains ill-defined.

Pharmacologic Choice. Most commonly, 20 to 30 ml of local anesthetic solution is injected via the interpleural needle or catheter. The most common local anesthetic concentrations used have been 0.25% or 0.5% bupivacaine.

Placement

Anatomy. The pleural space extends from the apex of the lung to the inferior reflection of the pleura at approximately L1. It also relates to the posterior and anterior mediastinal structures, as illustrated in Figure 32–1.

Position. The patient is most often turned to an oblique position, with the side to be blocked uppermost, as illustrated in Figure 32–2. The anesthesiologist stands to face the patient's back.

Needle Puncture. Once the patient is positioned properly and supported by a pillow, a skin wheal is raised immediately superior to the eighth rib in the seventh intercostal space, approximately 10 cm lateral to the midline. If a continuous technique is selected, a needle allowing passage of a catheter (often epidural) is selected. If a single injection technique is to be utilized, then a short, beveled needle of sufficient length to reach

Figure 32–1 Interpleural block—anatomy

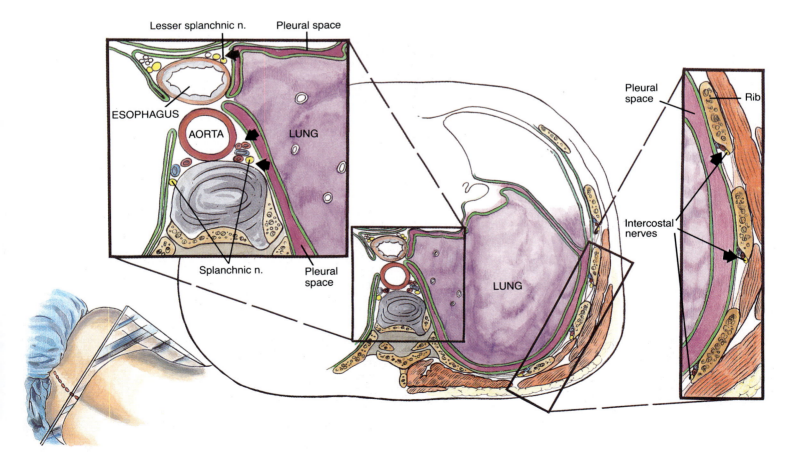

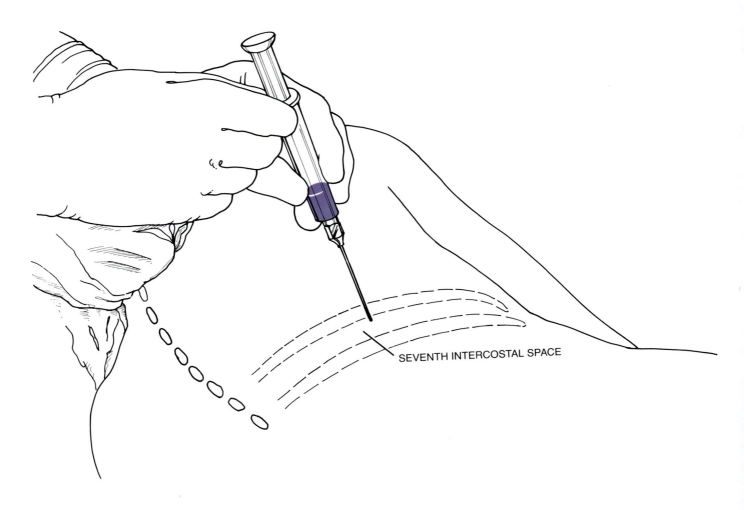

SEVENTH INTERCOSTAL SPACE

Figure 32–2 Interpleural block—position and technique

the pleural space can be used. (The proponents of this technique most often advocate intermittent injections via catheter; thus a single injection technique is unusual.) Prior to inserting the needle, a syringe containing approximately 2 ml of saline is inserted immediately superior to the eighth rib, utilizing a loss of resistance technique much like that used during epidural anesthesia. When the needle tip is in the pleural space, it will be very easy to inject local anesthetic solution.

Once the needle is in position, either the local anesthetic is injected, if it is to be a single shot technique, or a catheter is threaded through the needle. If a catheter is used, it should be threaded approximately 10 cm into the pleural space, taking care to minimize the volume of air entrained through the needle. The catheter is then taped in a position that will not interfere with the surgical

procedure, and local anesthetic is injected. Typically, from 20 to 30 ml of local anesthetic is injected, and, following this, the patient is rolled into the supine position to allow distribution of the local anesthetic.

Potential Problems. Although pneumothorax would seem to be associated with any technique that violates the pleural space, this seems to be an infrequent problem with interpleural anesthesia. Despite this observation, as time passes the true incidence of pneumothorax associated with this technique will become clearer. A second problem with interpleural anesthesia seems to be the unpredictable nature of analgesia accompanying what otherwise seems to be an acceptable technique. This may be a result of anesthesiologists' gaining experience with the technique, or perhaps it is the result of overzealous promotion of the technique.

Pearls

At this time, the mechanism behind interpleural anesthesia remains uncertain. As illustrated in Figure 32–1, one mechanism proposed for interpleural anesthesia is that the local anesthetic diffuses from the pleural space through the intercostal membrane to reach the intercostal nerves along the chest wall. A second mechanism is that the local anesthetic is distributed through the pleura and into the region of the posterior mediastinum, at which point local anesthetic provides visceral analgesia by contacting the greater, lesser, and least splanchnic nerves. When data become available, we will likely find interpleural anesthesia to be a combination of these two mechanisms, and perhaps others as well.

33

Lumbar Somatic Block

Perspective

Lumbar somatic block is often used to complement an anesthetic in which multiple intercostal nerve blocks have been used. Lumbar somatic block, together with intercostal nerve block, allows anesthesia for lower abdominal and even upper leg surgery. For example, lumbar somatic block of T12, L1, and L2 will cover most of the requirements for inguinal herniorrhaphy. Likewise, individual blocks of lumbar nerves (including blockade of T12 off the L1 spine) may allow differentiation of lower abdominal and postherniorrhaphy pain syndromes.

Patient Selection. Lumbar somatic block is often used in a pain clinic setting. However, some surgical patients, such as those undergoing herniorrhaphy, benefit from appropriate use of the block. In addition, although the frequency of flank incision for renal surgical procedures has decreased since the advent of lithotripsy, patients undergoing flank incisions are well managed with a combination of lower intercostal and lumbar somatic blockade and "light" general anesthesia.

Pharmacologic Selection. The local anesthetic choice for lumbar somatic block is limited only by the extent of additional blockade and concerns over systemic toxicity. If pinpoint diagnostic accuracy is essential for chronic pain syndromes, local anesthetic volumes as small as 1 to 2 ml are appropriate; if surgical anesthesia is desired, volumes of 5 to 7 ml per lumbar root are appropriate.

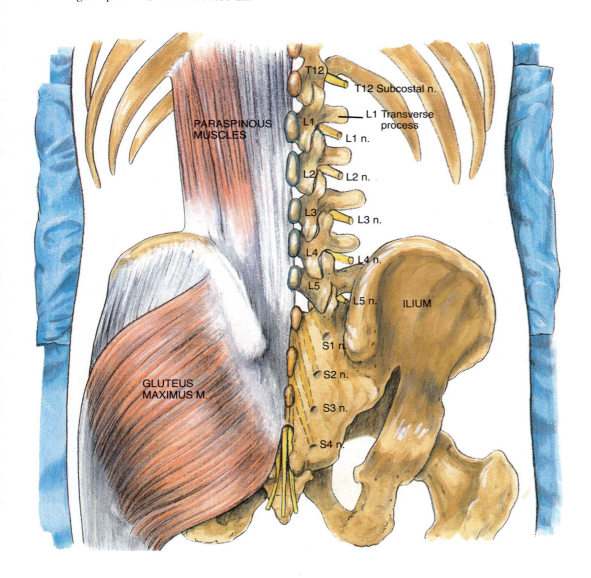

Figure 33–1 Lumbar somatic block— anatomy

Figure 33–2 Lumbar somatic block— anatomy

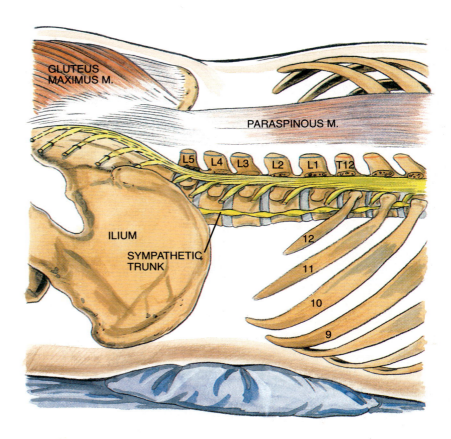

Placement

Anatomy. It is useful to conceptualize paravertebral lumbar somatic block as an intercostal block in miniature. Using this concept, the short vertebral transverse process (a "rudimentary rib") becomes the principal focus and landmark for needle position. Each lumbar somatic nerve leaves the vertebral foramina slightly caudal and ventral to the transverse process of its respective vertebral level (Fig. 33–1).

As Figure 33–2 illustrates, from the intervertebral foramina the lumbar somatic nerves angle caudad and anteriorly and, in this process, pass anterior to the lateral extent of the transverse process of the next lower vertebral body (Fig. 33–1). For example, as the L1 somatic root leaves its intervertebral foramen, its route places it immediately anterior at the lateral border of the L2 transverse process. Similarly, the T12 somatic root (a subcostal nerve) is found immediately anterior at the lateral extent of the L1 transverse process.

Returning to the intercostal nerve analogy, each lumbar nerve gives off an immediate

posterior branch to the paravertebral muscles and skin of the back. Again, as with intercostal nerve anatomy, the lumbar somatic also receives white rami communicantes from the upper two or three lumbar nerves, as well as giving rise to gray rami communicantes to all lumbar somatic nerves. Following these connections to the sympathetic nervous system, the main somatic nerve then passes directly into the psoas major muscle or comes to lie in a plane between the psoas and quadratus lumborum muscles. Here the nerves intertwine to form the lumbar plexus. Figure 33–3 highlights this cross-sectional anatomy. Figure 33–4 illustrates the cutaneous distribution of the lumbar somatic nerves.

Position. The concept that this block is similar to an intercostal nerve block carries through to the actual performance of the technique. The most advantageous position is to have the patient prone with a pillow under the lower abdomen to reduce lumbar lordosis. Skin markings are made as illustrated in Figure 33–5—that is, the lumbar spinous process of each vertebra corresponding to roots to be blocked is identified and marked.

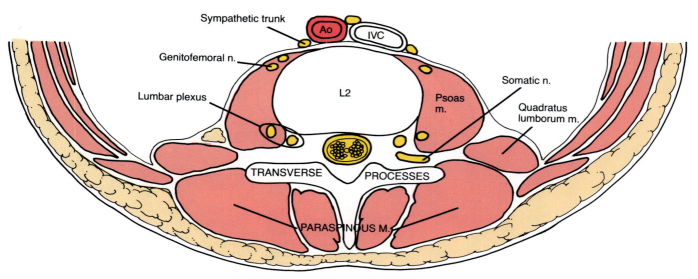

Figure 33–3 Lumbar somatic block—cross-sectional anatomy

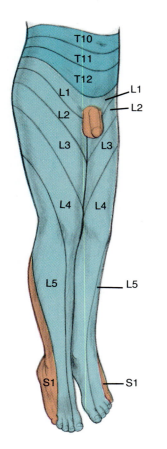

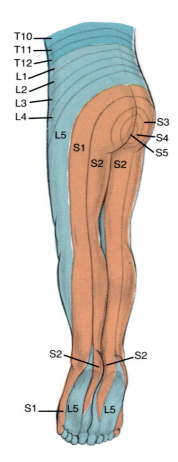

Figure 33–4 Lumbar somatic block—dermatomal anatomy

Figure 33–5 Lumbar somatic block—surface anatomy

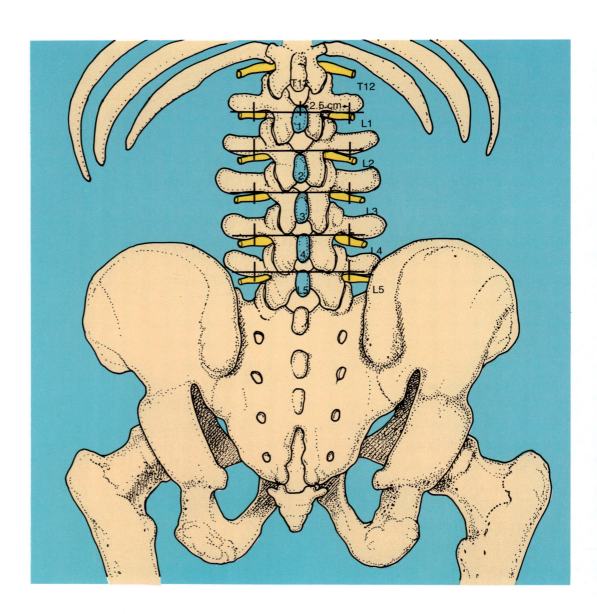

Then, from the cephalic edge of each of these lumbar posterior spines, lines are drawn horizontally and marks placed on the lines 2.5 to 3 cm from the midline. The anatomic concept behind these markings is that the cephalic edge of each lumbar posterior spine is approximately on the same horizontal plane as its own vertebral transverse process. Skin wheals are then made at the site 2.5 to 3 cm from the midline on the lines overlying the lower edge of the transverse process. Through the skin wheals an 8-cm, 22-gauge needle is inserted in a vertical plane without a syringe attached (Fig. 33–6). As the needle is advanced, it will contact the transverse process at a depth of 3 to 5 cm in the aver-

age adult *(needle position 1)*. Failure to contact the transverse processes at that depth implies that the needle has passed between the two transverse processes.

To contact bone, a repeat insertion is made through the same skin wheal, but with a slight cephalic angulation of the needle. Once the transverse process has been identified, the needle tip is withdrawn to a subcutaneous location before being reinserted to pass just caudal to the previously identified transverse process. This allows blockade of the lumbar root corresponding to the same lumbar vertebra. The needle is reinserted just cephalic to the corresponding transverse process in order to block the lumbar root one

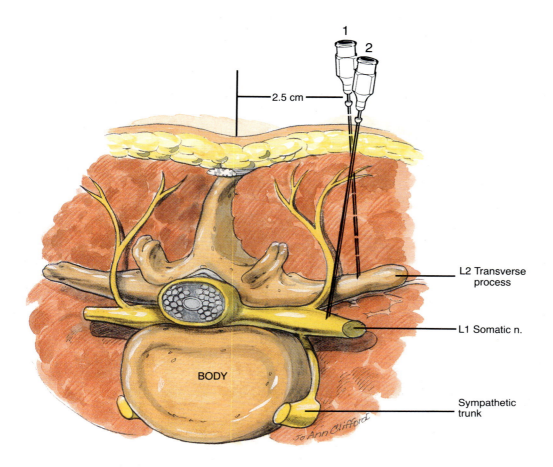

Figure 33—6 Lumbar somatic block—technique

1
2

2.5 cm

L2 Transverse process

L1 Somatic n.

BODY

Sympathetic trunk

JoAnnClifford

segment more cephalic. As you "slide" the needle off and past the transverse process, the needle should be advanced approximately the thickness of the transverse process, or approximately 1 to 2 cm, after contact with bone is lost (needle position 2). This will place the tip in the plane immediately anterior to the transverse process. When final needle position has been established, approximately 5 ml of local anesthetic solution is injected. The process should be repeated at each site at which local anesthetic blockade is desired.

Potential Problems. Since the lumbar roots are in close proximity to other centroneuraxis structures, keep in mind that epidural and subarachnoid anesthesia has been produced following attempts at lumbar somatic block. It is most likely that in these cases the needle was angled medially during insertion rather than being maintained in a parasagittal plane. Likewise, because of the proximity of the sympathetic ganglion to the lumbar roots, if needles are inserted too deeply the

volume of local anesthetic solution injected is often enough to cause lumbar sympathetic blockade. If that happens, a decrease in blood pressure similar to that seen during low spinal anesthesia may result.

Pearls

Blockade of the 12th thoracic nerve is effectively carried out by blocking the root immediately superior to the L1 transverse process. This method is often preferable to attempts to block it like an intercostal nerve at the angle of the ribs. If these blocks are used for herniorrhaphy procedures, be sure to recognize that a long-acting local anesthetic of sufficient concentration to produce motor blockade may limit patients from walking normally for a number of hours, since some weakness of the hip flexors may be produced with blockade of L1 and L2 roots.

34

Inguinal Block

Perspective

Inguinal blockade is primarily a technique of peripheral blockade for inguinal herniorrhaphy.

Patient Selection. Increasing numbers of patients are undergoing inguinal herniorrhaphy as outpatients; thus, this block may be incorporated in most practices.

Pharmacologic Choice. As with many of the peripheral regional blocks, motor blockade is not essential for success with inguinal block. Therefore, lower concentrations of intermediate- to long-acting local anesthetics can be chosen. For example, 1% lidocaine or 1% mepivacaine is appropriate, as is 0.25% bupivacaine. The anesthetist should be aware that it is often necessary to supplement inguinal block intraoperatively by injection in the vi-

cinity of the spermatic cord by the surgeon. Therefore, the volume of local anesthetic used during the initial block should not preclude additional intraoperative injection.

Placement

Anatomy. Innervation of the inguinal region arises from the distal extensions of the more cephalic lumbar plexus nerves—that is, the iliohypogastric and ilioinguinal nerves, which have their origin from the first lumbar nerve, and the genitofemoral nerve, which has its origin from the first and second lumbar nerves (Fig. 34–1). These peripheral extensions of the lumbar plexus and the 12th thoracic nerve follow a circular course that is influenced by the bowl-like shape of the ili-

Figure 34–1 Inguinal block—anatomy

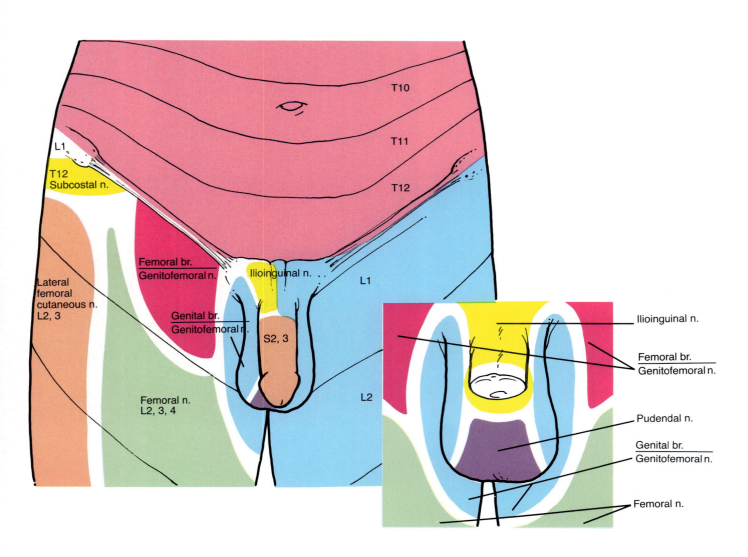

um. As these nerves course anteriorly, as illustrated in Figure 34–2, they pass near an important landmark for the block, the anterior superior iliac spine. In the vicinity of the anterior superior iliac spine, the 12th thoracic and iliohypogastric nerves lie between the internal and external oblique muscles. The ilioinguinal nerve lies between the transversus abdominis muscle and the internal oblique muscle initially and then penetrates the internal oblique muscle some distance medial to the anterior superior spine. All these nerves continue anterior medially and become superficial as they terminate in the skin and muscles of the inguinal region (Fig. 34–3). As also shown in Figure 34–3, the genitofemoral nerve follows a different course, and it is this nerve that must often be supple-

mented intraoperatively to make this regional block effective for inguinal herniorraphy.

Position. This block can be carried out with the patient in the supine position and the anesthesiologist at the patient's side in a position to utilize the anterosuperior iliac spine as a landmark.

Needle Puncture. While the patient is in the supine position, the anterosuperior iliac spine should be marked. Another mark should be made approximately 3 cm medial and inferior to the anterosuperior iliac spine. A skin wheal is created, and an 8-cm, 22-gauge needle is inserted in a cephalolateral direction *(needle position 1)* to contact the inner surface of the ilium, as illustrated in Figure 34–4. Ten milliliters of local anesthetic solution is injected as the needle is slowly

Figure 34–2 Inguinal block—anatomy

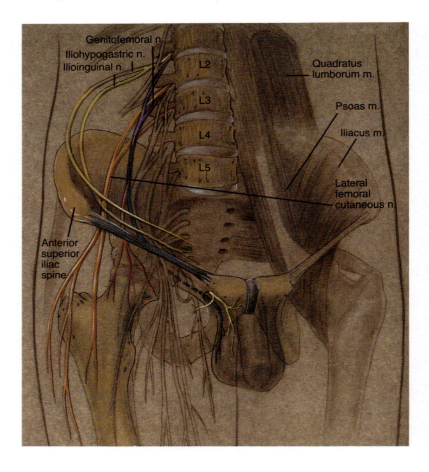

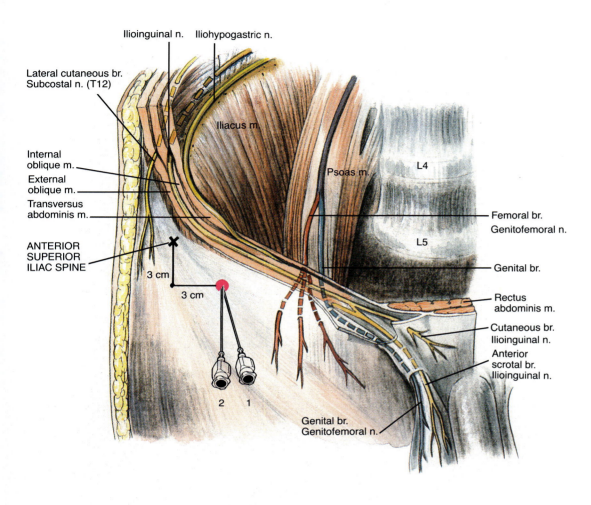

Ilioinguinal n.   Iliohypogastric n.

Lateral cutaneous br.
Subcostal n. (T12)

Iliacus m.

Internal
oblique m.

External
oblique m.

Transversus
abdominis m.

ANTERIOR
SUPERIOR
ILIAC SPINE

3 cm

3 cm

2   1

Psoas m.

L4

L5

Femoral br.
Genitofemoral n.

Genital br.

Rectus
abdominis m.

Cutaneous br.
Ilioinguinal n.

Anterior
scrotal br.
Ilioinguinal n.

Genital br.
Genitofemoral n.

Figure 34–3 Inguinal block—anatomy and technique

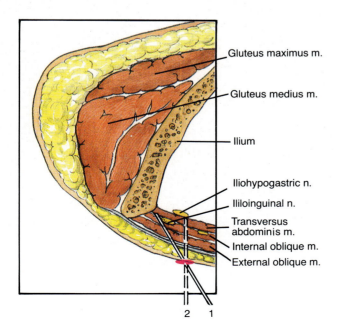

Gluteus maximus m.

Gluteus medius m.

Ilium

Iliohypogastric n.

Ililoinguinal n.

Transversus
abdominis m.

Internal oblique m.

External oblique m.

2   1

Figure 34–4 Inguinal block—cross-sectional anatomy and technique

withdrawn through the layers of the abdominal wall. The needle should then be reinserted at a steeper angle to insure penetration of all three abdominal muscle layers *(needle position 2)*. Again, the injection is repeated as the needle is withdrawn. In patients who are heavily muscled or obese, a third injection may be necessary at an even steeper angle. From the previously placed skin wheal, extension of the injection is made toward the umbilicus, creating a subcutaneous field block. This process is repeated from umbilicus to pubis (Fig. 34–5). Again, consideration that the surgeon will need to inject additional local anesthetic into the cord should be kept in mind, so that this necessary part of the block can be added intraoperatively without concern over local anesthetic systemic toxicity.

Potential Problems. This block is primarily a superficial block and is associated with few major complications. Some proponents of this technique advocate injecting in the region of the inguinal canal and spermatic cord preoperatively. A potential problem with this additional injection is that hematoma formation is possible in the region of the cord. This does not cause harm to the patient; however, the surgeon may find it very difficult to perform an adequate surgical dissection.

Pearls

The key to utilizing this block successfully is combining adequate sedation with a systematic method of injecting local anesthetic near the iliac crest. The "system" should be established to assure that the anesthetic has been deposited at all body wall levels.

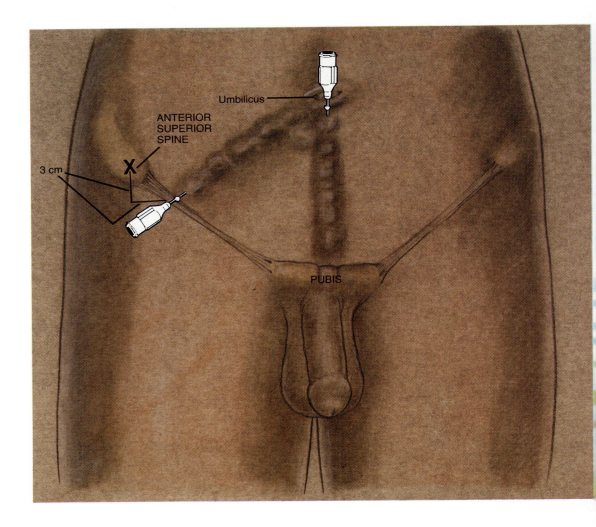

Figure 34–5 Inguinal block—infiltration technique

35

Lumbar Sympathetic Block

Perspective

Lumbar sympathetic blocks are typically carried out to (1) improve blood flow to the lower extremities or (2) provide pain relief to lower extremities.

Patient Selection. Patients requiring lumbar sympathetic blockade can be divided into two primary groups: (1) those requiring sympathetic blockade on the basis of ischemic vascular disease to the lower extremities (these patients are often older), and (2) patients requiring the block for diagnosis or treatment of reflex sympathetic dystrophy of the lower extremities (these patients will have a much wider spectrum of ages).

Pharmacologic Choice. Blockade of the sympathetic nervous system can be performed with lower concentrations of local anesthetics than almost any other regional blocks. For example, 0.5% lidocaine or 0.125% or 0.25% bupivacaine is an appropriate choice.

Placement

Anatomy. The lumbar sympathetic chain, with its accompanying ganglia, is located in the fascial plane immediately anterolateral to the lumbar vertebral bodies (Fig. 35–1). The sympathetic chain is separated from the somatic nerves by the psoas muscle and fascia. The lumbar regions L1, L2, and sometimes L3 provide white rami communicantes to the sympathetic chain, while all five lumbar vertebrae are associated with gray rami communicantes. These rami are longer in the lumbar region than they are in the thoracic region. This is anatomically important, since it allows needle placement nearer the anterolateral border of the vertebral body in the lumbar region. Conceptually, the anatomy important to anesthesiologists for lumbar sympathetic nerve block is also the anatomy important for celiac plexus nerve block.

Position. My experience suggests that lumbar sympathetic nerve block is most effectively carried out in a manner similar to that for celiac plexus block. The patient should be in a prone position with a pillow under the mid-abdomen to help reduce lumbar lordosis. (In spite of this recommendation, many continue to successfully use the lateral position.)

Needle Puncture. Most experienced anesthesiologists now carry out this block through a single needle. This is possible, since placing the needle tip at the anterolateral border of the second or third lumbar vertebral body allows spread of local anesthetic solution along the fascial plane enveloping the sympathetic chain. As an example, the second lumbar vertebral spine is identified and a mark made lateral to it in the horizontal plane, 7 to 9 cm from the midline, as illustrated in Figure 35–2. A skin wheal is raised, and a 15-cm, 20- or 22-gauge needle is directed in the horizontal plane at an angle of 30° to 45° from a vertical plane through the patient's midline and inserted until it

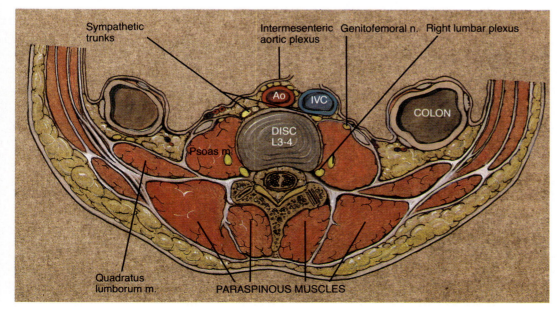

Sympathetic trunks — Intermesenteric aortic plexus — Genitofemoral n. — Right lumbar plexus — Ao — IVC — COLON — DISC L3-4 — Psoas m. — Quadratus lumborum m. — PARASPINOUS MUSCLES

Figure 35–1 Lumbar sympathetic block—cross-sectional anatomy

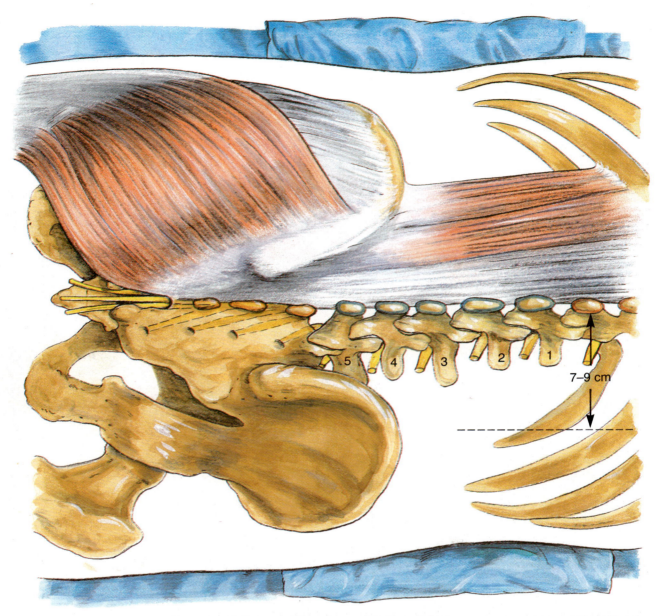

7–9 cm

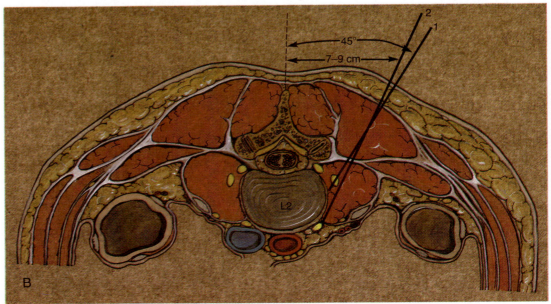

Figure 35–2 Lumbar sympathetic block—surface *(A)* and cross-sectional *(B)* technique

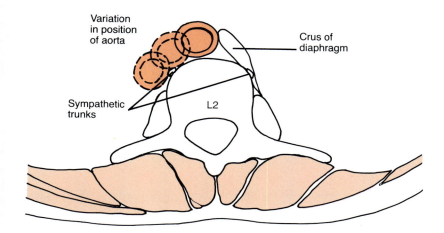

Variation
in position
of aorta

Crus of
diaphragm

Sympathetic
trunks

L2

Figure 35–3 Lumbar sympathetic block—aortic variation

contacts the lateral aspect of the L2 vertebral body. If it comes into contact at a more superficial level with the vertebral transverse process (at only 3 to 5 cm), simply redirect the needle in a cephalic or caudal manner to avoid the transverse process. The vertebral body will usually be located at a depth of 7 to 12 cm.

Once the needle's position on the lateral aspect of the vertebral body is certain, the needle is withdrawn and redirected at a steeper angle to slide off the anterolateral surface of L2. Once again, it is emphasized that this needle insertion and redirection are almost identical to those described for celiac plexus block. For lumbar sympathetic blockade, once the needle is in position, approximately 15 to 20 ml of local anesthetic solution is injected through this single needle. With proper needle tip position, this volume will allow spread along the axis of the sympathetic chain.

Potential Problems. As illustrated in Figure 35–3, a potential problem from lumbar sympathetic block is puncture of the aorta. It is emphasized that most often this results in no sequelae. Nevertheless, anesthetists should be aware that the position of the aorta in relationship to the vertebral body ranges from an anterolateral position to a midline position. This concept also needs to be kept in mind during celiac plexus blockade. Because of the needle direction toward centroneuraxis structures, be aware that both epidural and spinal block can result from errantly placed needles. Also, when using neurolytic agents, be aware that "spill over" on to lumbar roots is a possibility, although rare.

Pearls

Few regional blocks are as similar as lumbar sympathetic blockade and celiac plexus block. Thus, if the concepts behind one technique are understood, it is quite easy to translate that anatomic understanding into successful performance of the other. Adequate sedation for placing the needle against the lateral portion of the second lumbar vertebra is also essential for patient—and thus anesthesiolgist—satisfaction.

36

Celiac Plexus Block

Figure 36–4 Celiac plexus block—functional anatomy

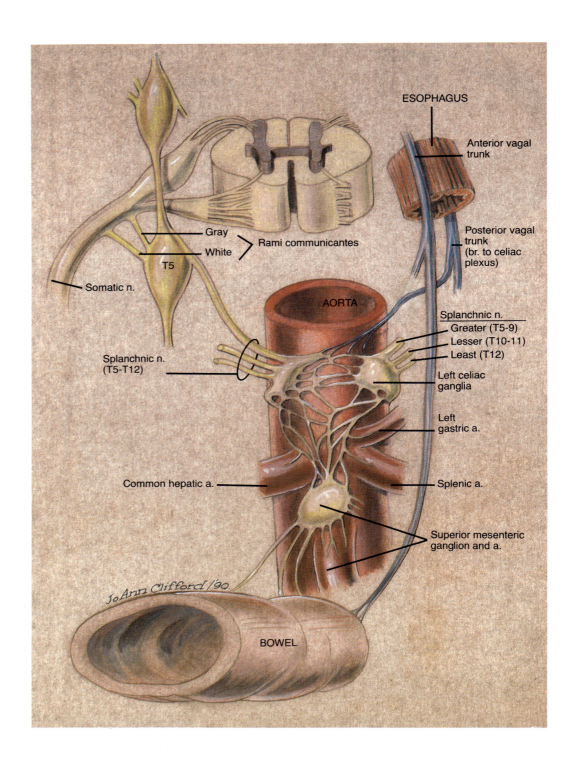

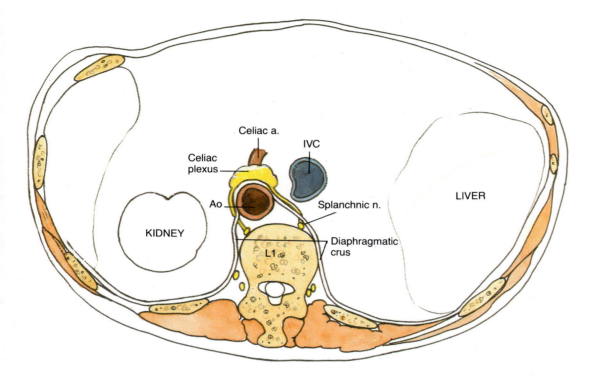

Figure 36–5 Celiac plexus block—cross-sectional magnetic resonance imaging anatomy—interpretation

Figure 36–6 Celiac plexus block—cross-sectional magnetic resonance anatomy—scan

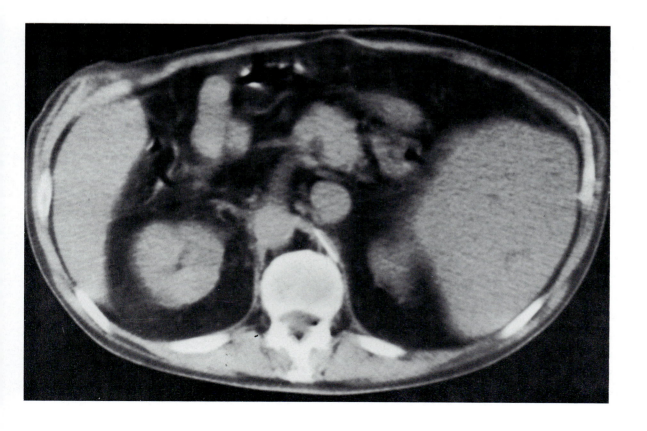

Figure 36–7 Celiac plexus block—retro- and anterocrural relationships

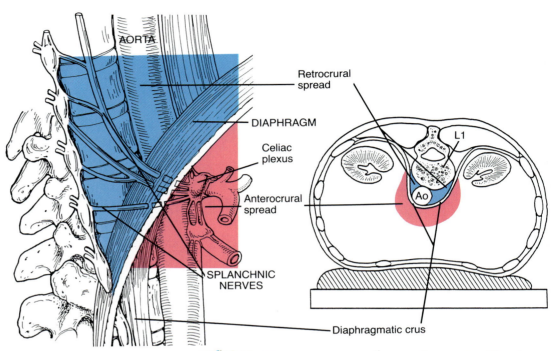

Figure 36–8 Celiac plexus block—surface anatomy and markings

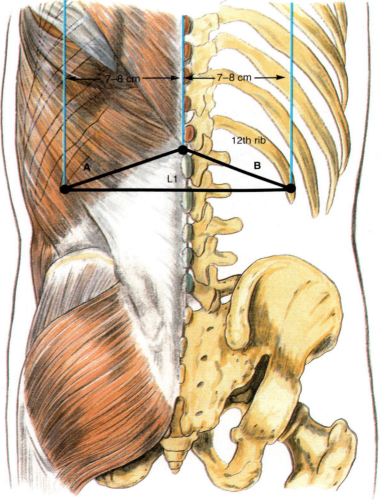

erally. Another mark should be placed in the midline between the 12th thoracic and 1st lumbar vertebral spines. By drawing lines between the three marks, a flat isosceles triangle is created. The equal sides of this triangle (A and B) serve as directional guides for the bilaterally placed needles.

Skin wheals should then be raised on the marks immediately below the twelfth rib, and a 12- to 15-cm, 20-gauge needle is inserted without the syringe attached, as shown in Figure 36–9. The needle is inserted 45° off the plane of the "table top," directed at the space between T12 and L1 vertebral spines. This placement will allow contact with L1 vertebral body at a depth of 7 to 9 cm. If bony contact is made at a more superficial level, it is likely that a vertebral transverse process has been contacted.

When the vertebral body is confidently identified, the needle is withdrawn to a subcutaneous level and the angle increased to allow the tip to pass the lateral border of the vertebral body. On the left side (the side of the aorta), once the needle passes off the vertebral body, it should be inserted an additional 1.5 to 2 cm or until the aortic wall is identified by pulsations transmitted via the length of the needle. On the right side, the needle can be inserted from 2 to 3 cm after it walks off the vertebral body. A help in inserting the needles to the proper depth is to insert the left needle first, since it can be advanced slowly until one's sensitive finger tips (as illustrated in Figure 36–10) appreciate the aortic pulsations being transmitted up the needle shaft. When this aortic depth is identified, the right-sided needle can then be inserted and readily advanced to a slightly deeper level.

Prior to the injection of local anesthetic or neurolytic agent, the needle should be carefully examined for leakage of blood, urine, or cerebrospinal fluid. If the needle is misplaced, the leakage of these fluids should be spontaneous. Injection of local anesthetic solution through the needle should be similar to that experienced when an epidural needle is

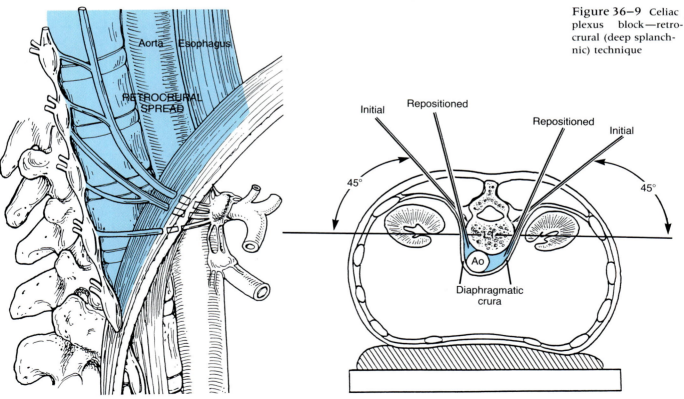

Figure 36–9 Celiac plexus block—retrocrural (deep splanchnic) technique

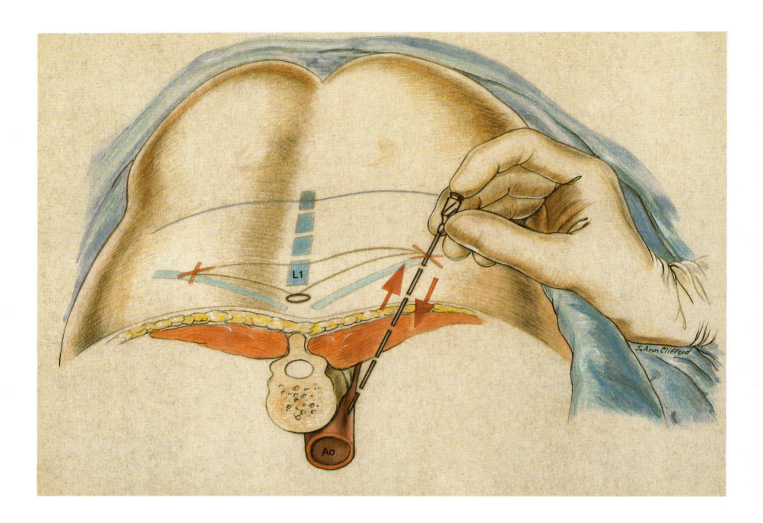

Figure 36—10 Celiac plexus block—finger as "pressure transducer" technique

properly placed. There should be very little resistance to injection if a 20-gauge needle is correctly placed in the retrocrural area.

Needle Puncture—Anterocrural Method. The second basic method of celiac plexus blockade is to use an anterocrural approach, which results in the needle tip being placed anterior to the crus of the diaphragm on the right side, as illustrated in Figure 36—11. To carry out this block, all the foregoing steps are the same, except that the paramedian line on the right is drawn 5 to 6 cm off the midline rather than 7 to 8 cm as with the classic retrocrural approach. The needle is again inserted to strike the vertebral body. Often an angle larger than 45° is necessary to contact the vertebral body initially. When the vertebral body is contacted, the needle is

withdrawn and redirected until it walks off the anterolateral edge of the vertebral body. To place an anterocrural needle properly, radiographic assistance is necessary. Commonly, to place the needle tip anterior to the crus of the diaphragm requires 10 to 13 cm of needle insertion. It is helpful to use a supplementary imaging technique for the transcrural approach, since passage of the needle tip through the crus of the diaphragm is difficult to appreciate by palpation unless a transaortic method similar to Ischia is used. Once the needle tip is in position anterior to the crus of the diaphragm, local anesthetic solution is injected through the single right-sided needle.

Potential Problems. The location of the celiac plexus near the centroneuraxis allows de-

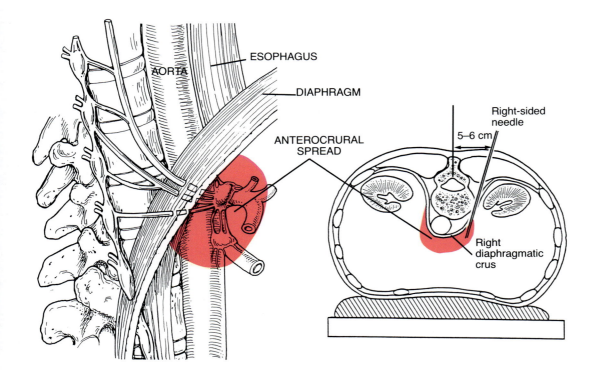

ESOPHAGUS

AORTA

DIAPHRAGM

ANTEROCRURAL
SPREAD

Right-sided
needle

5–6 cm

Right
diaphragmatic
crus

Figure 36–11 Celiac plexus block—anterocrural technique

velopment of epidural or spinal anesthesia with the technique. Additionally, because of the close relationship of the celiac plexus to the aorta, aortic puncture is encountered in approximately one third of patients. Nevertheless, this rarely should result in serious problems. As in a lumbar sympathetic blockade, the placement of the needle tip with celiac block can allow tracking of local anesthetic or neurolytic solution in the region of the lumbar roots, although this also appears to be infrequent.

Pearls

To understand celiac plexus block fully, one should be familiar with the concept of retrocrural and anterocrural blockade. This understanding helps anesthesiologists develop a three-dimensional "feel" for location of needle tip. With the patient in the prone position, adequate sedation can also be administered and will go a long way toward making the anesthesiologist and the patient comfortable during plexus blockade.

37

Centroneuraxis Anatomy

Centroneuraxis blocks—spinal, epidural, and caudal—are the most widely used regional blocks. The main reasons for their popularity are that the blocks have well-defined endpoints, and that the anesthesiologist can produce blockade reliably with a single injection. The first step in being able to use centroneuraxis blocks effectively is to develop an understanding of centroneuraxis anatomy.

As illustrated in Figure 37–1, to understand centroneuraxis anatomy it is necessary to develop a concept of the relationship between surface and bony anatomy pertinent to centroneuraxis structures. Beginning cephalically, the spine of the seventh cervical vertebra, the vertebral prominence, is the most prominent midline structure at the base of the neck. A line drawn between the lower borders of the scapula will cross the vertebral axis at approximately the T7 spine. The lower extent of the spinal cord, the conus medullaris, ends in the adult at approximately L1. (In the infant the conus medullaris may extend to L3.) The line between the iliac crests, Tuffier's line, most often crosses through the L4 spine. A line drawn between the posterior superior iliac spines identifies the level of the second sacral vertebra and the distal extent of the dural sac containing cerebrospinal fluid (CSF).

The 33 vertebrae from C1 to the tip of the coccyx have a number of common features, as well as differences, which should be highlighted. Each vertebra contains a spinous process that is joined to the lamina from which a transverse process extends laterally into both lamina and pedicle. The pedicle joins this posterior assembly to the vertebral body, which relates to the neighboring vertebral bodies through both superior and inferior facet joints (Fig. 37–2). Figure 37–3 outlines the general relationship with these structures at levels that correspond to common sites for cervical, thoracic, and lumbar punctures of the centroneuraxis.

The lateral, oblique and posterior views highlight two features of bony anatomy that need emphasis. First, in the cervical and lumbar vertebrae, the spinous process assumes a more horizontal orientation than does the spinous process in the midthoracic region. The caudal angulation of the spinous process in the midthoracic region highlights why needle puncture of the centroneuraxis structures in this area requires a more cephalic needle angulation. Conversely, in both the cervical and lumbar regions, more direct (perpendicular) needle angulation is possible in reaching centroneuraxis structures. The

Figure 37–1 Centroneuraxis anatomy—surface relationships

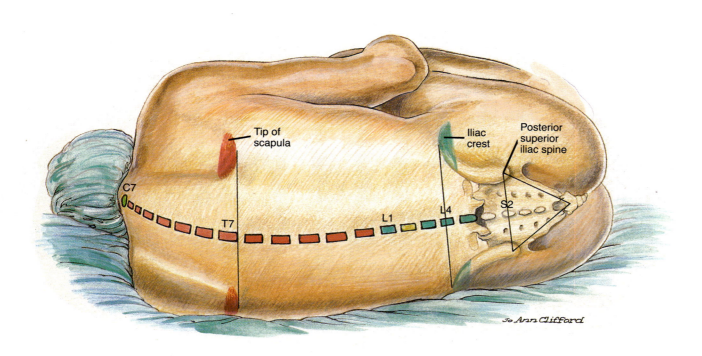

Figure 37–2 Centroneuraxis anatomy—lumbar vertebral anatomy

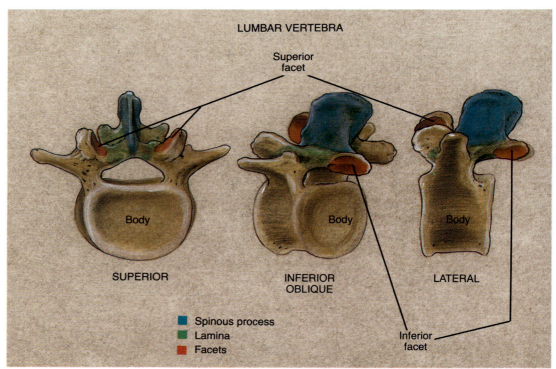

Figure 37–3 Centroneuraxis anatomy—vertebral column relationships

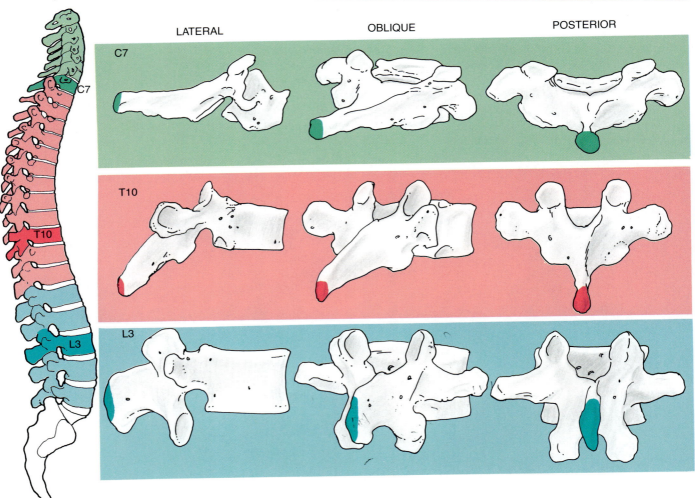

gulation of the lamina immediately lateral to the spinous process in the three regions. As illustrated by the black line in the lateral view of the vertebral bodies, from cephalad to caudad the vertebral laminae become more vertical in orientation. Both these features will become important as an understanding is developed of "walking" needles off the lamina into the desired centroneuraxis locations.

In addition to the bony relationships of the vertebral bodies, there are important ligamentous relationships. As illustrated in Figure 37–4, defining the posterior limit of the epidural space is the ligamentum flavum, or "yellow ligament." This ligament extends from the foramen magnum to the sacral hiatus. Although classically portrayed as a single ligament, it is really composed of two ligamenta flava, the right and the left, which join in the midline. The ligamentum flavum is not uniform from skull to sacrum, nor even within an intervertebral space. Within an individual intervertebral space, the ligamentum flavum is thicker caudally than cephalically and thicker in the midline than on its lateral borders. Immediately posterior to the ligamentum flavum are either lamina and spinous processes of vertebral bodies, or the interspinous ligament. Extending from the

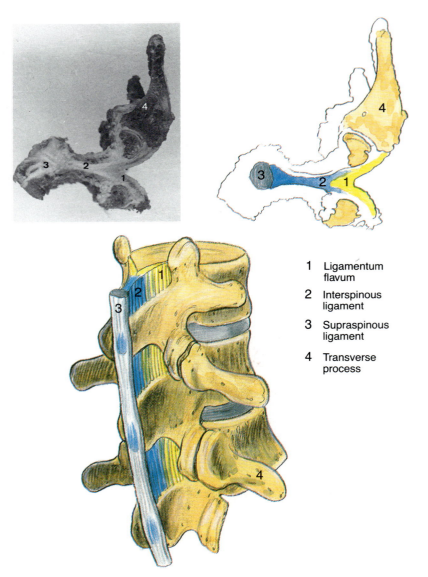

Figure 37–4 Centroneuraxis anatomy—lumbar vertebral ligaments (photograph with permission of Zarzur and Elsevier)

1 Ligamentum flavum

2 Interspinous ligament

3 Supraspinous ligament

4 Transverse process

interspinous ligament. Extending from the external occipital protuberance to the coccyx posterior to these structures is the supraspinous ligament, which joins the vertebral spines.

Most centroneuraxis blocks are performed in the lumbar region. Figures 37–5, 37–6, and 37–7 illustrate the anatomy in the poste-

rior, lateral, and horizontal planes, respectively. Surrounding the spinal cord in the bony vertebral column are three membranes. From immediate overlay of the cord to the periphery, these are the pia mater, arachnoid mater, and dura mater. The *pia mater* is a highly vascular membrane that closely invests the spinal cord. The *arachnoid mater* is a

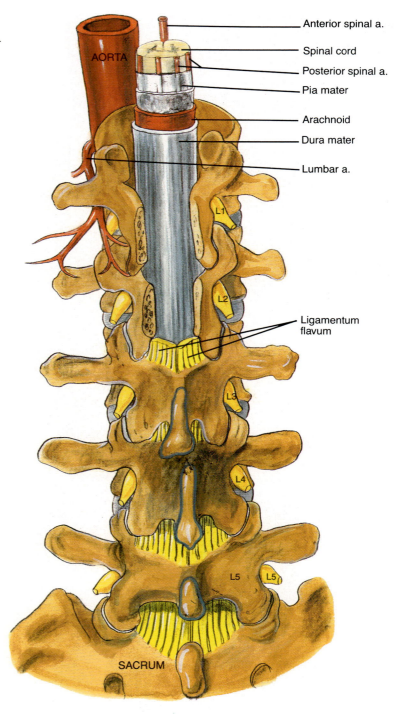

Figure 37–5 Centroneuraxis anatomy—lumbar detail—posterior

Anterior spinal a.

Spinal cord

Posterior spinal a.

Pia mater

Arachnoid

Dura mater

Lumbar a.

Ligamentum flavum

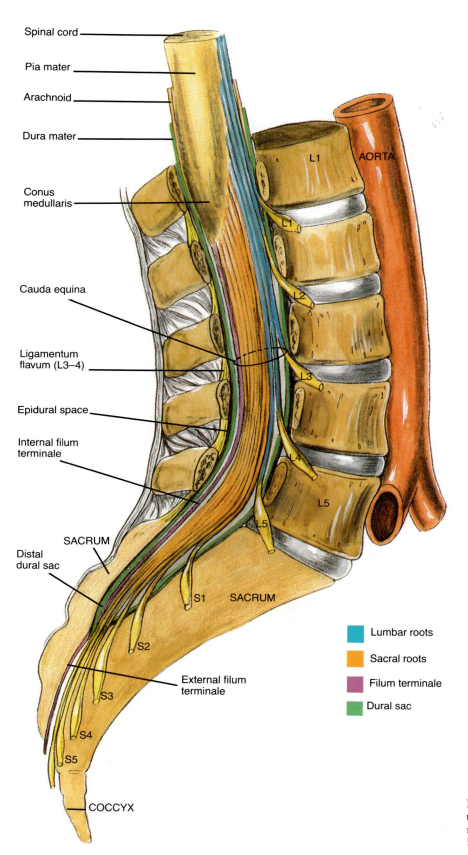

Spinal cord

Pia mater

Arachnoid

Dura mater

Conus medullaris

Cauda equina

Ligamentum flavum (L3–4)

Epidural space

Internal filum terminale

SACRUM

Distal dural sac

External filum terminale

COCCYX

L1

AORTA

L1

L2

L3

L4

L5

L5

S1

SACRUM

S2

S3

S4

S5

Lumbar roots

Sacral roots

Filum terminale

Dural sac

Figure 37–6 Centroneuraxis anatomy—lumbar detail—lateral

Figure 37—7 Centroneuraxis anatomy—lumbar detail—cross-sectional

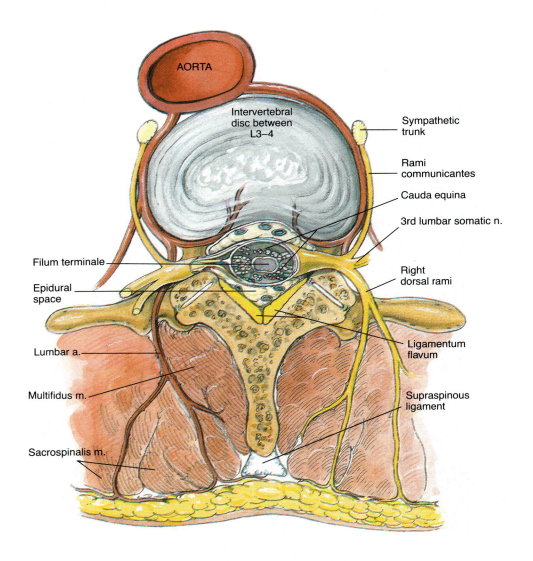

AORTA

Intervertebral disc between L3–4

Sympathetic trunk

Rami communicantes

Cauda equina

3rd lumbar somatic n.

Filum terminale

Epidural space

Right dorsal rami

Lumbar a.

Ligamentum flavum

Multifidus m.

Supraspinous ligament

Sacrospinalis m.

delicate, nonvascular membrane closely attached to the outermost layer, the dura. Between the pia and arachnoid is the space of interest in spinal anesthesia, the subarachnoid space. In this space are the CSF, spinal nerves, a trabecular network between the two membranes, blood vessels that supply the spinal cord, and the lateral extensions of the pia mater, the dentate ligaments. These dentate ligaments supply lateral support from the spinal cord to the dura mater and may become important conceptually when unilateral or patchy spinal anesthesia results from what appears to be an adequate technical block. The third and outermost membrane in the spinal canal is the longitudinally organized fibroelastic membrane called the *dura mater* (or theca). This layer is the direct extension of the cranial dura mater and extends

as spinal dura mater from the foramen magnum to S2, where the filum terminale (an extension of the pia mater beginning at the conus medullaris) blends with the periosteum on the coccyx (Fig. 37–6). There is a potential space between the dura mater and the arachnoid, the subdural space, which contains only small amounts of serous fluid to allow the dura and arachnoid to move over each other. This space is not intentionally utilized by anesthesiologists, though injection into it during spinal anesthesia may explain the occasional "failed" spinal anesthetic and the rare "total spinal" following epidural anesthesia, when there was no indication of errant injection of the local anesthetic into the CSF.

Surrounding the dura mater, and in its posterior extent immediately anterior to the ligamentum flavum, is another space effectively used by anesthesiologists, the epidural space. The spinal epidural space extends from the foramen magnum to the sacral hiatus and surrounds the dura mater anteriorly, laterally, and, more useful, posteriorly. Contents of the epidural space include the nerve roots that traverse it from the intervertebral foramina to the peripheral locations, as well as fat, areolar tissue, lymphatics, and blood vessels, which include the well-organized venous plexus of Batson.

Through advances in epiduroscopy and epidurography, the occasionally unilateral anesthesia that follows apparently adequate epidural technique has been explained anatomically. An almost universal appearance of a dorsomedian connective tissue band in the midline of the epidural space has been noted with these techniques as well as with anatomic dissection.

Anatomy important during caudal anesthesia is an extension of epidural anatomy, although the frequent variations in sacral anatomy deserve emphasis. The sacrum results from the fusion of the five sacral vertebrae, whereas the sacral hiatus results from the failure of the laminae of S5 and usually part of S4 to fuse in the midline. The sacral hiatus results in a variably shaped and sized, inverted **V**-shaped bony defect, covered by the posterior sacrococcygeal ligament that is a functional counterpart to the ligamentum flavum (Fig. 37–8). The hiatus may be identified by locating the sacral cornu (remnants of the S5 articular processes). This bony defect allows percutaneous access to the sacral canal, although the frequent anatomic variation of the sacral hiatus can make caudal block confusing. The sacral canal is functionally the distal extent of the epidural space, and from this canal the pelvic sacral foramina open ventrally toward the ischial rectal fossa, while the dorsal sacral foramina open in a posterior direction (Fig. 37–8). In the sacral canal, the nerves of the cauda equina continue their routes until they exit via their respective vertebral foramina. Once again, the dural sac continues to the level of S2, or the line joining the posterior superior spines.

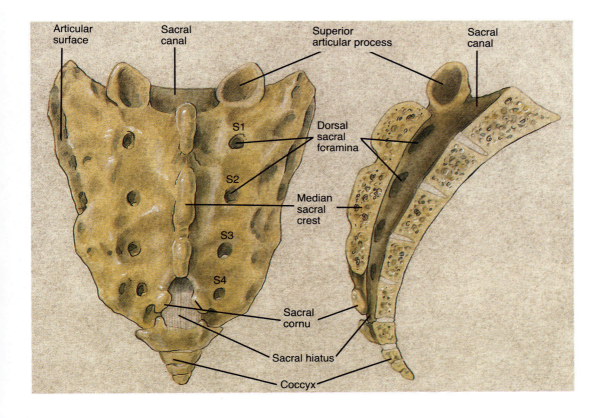

Figure 37–8 Centroneuraxis anatomy—sacrum

38

Spinal Block

Perspective

Spinal anesthesia is unparalleled in the way a small mass of drug, virtually devoid of systemic pharmacologic effect, can produce profound, reproducible surgical anesthesia. Further, by altering the small mass of drug, very different spinal anesthetics can be produced. Low spinal anesthesia, a block below T10, carries a different physiologic impact than does a block performed to produce higher spinal anesthesia (greater than T5). The block is unexcelled for lower abdominal or lower extremity surgical procedures. However, for operations in the mid- to upper abdomen, "light" general anesthesia may have to supplement the spinal block. This is because stimulation of the diaphragm during upper abdominal procedures often causes patients some discomfort. The area is difficult to block completely through high spinal anesthesia, since to do so requires blockade of the phrenic nerve.

Patient Selection. Patient selection for spinal anesthesia often places too much emphasis on a side effect of the technique—namely, spinal headache—than on the applicability of the technique for a given patient. It is clear that the incidence of spinal headache increases with decreasing age and female gender; however, with proper technique and selection of needle size, the incidence of headache should not preclude the use of spinal anesthesia in young, healthy patients if the block has advantages over epidural anesthesia. Almost any patient who is to have a lower extremity operation is a candidate for spinal anesthesia, as are most patients scheduled for lower abdominal surgery, such as inguinal herniorrhaphy and gynecologic, urologic, and obstetric procedures.

Pharmacologic Choice. In the United States, three local anesthetics are commonly used to produce spinal anesthesia: lidocaine, tetracaine, and bupivacaine. Lidocaine is a short- to intermediate-acting spinal drug; tetracaine and bupivacaine provide intermediate to long duration block. Lidocaine, without epinephrine, is often chosen for procedures that can be completed in 1 hour or less. The mixture most commonly used is a 5% solution in 7.5% dextrose. When epinephrine (0.2 mg) is added to lidocaine, the useful length of clinical anesthesia in the lower abdomen and lower extremities is approximately 90 minutes. Tetracaine is packaged as both niphanoid crystals (20 mg) and as a 1% solution (2 ml total). When dextrose is added to make tetracaine hyperbaric, the drug generally produces effective clinical anesthesia for procedures of up to 1.5 to 2 hours in the plain form, for up to 2 to 3 hours when epinephrine (0.2 mg) is added, and up to 5 hours for lower extremity procedures when phenylephrine (5 mg) is added as a vasoconstrictor. Bupivacaine spinal anesthesia is commonly carried out with 0.5% or 0.75% solution, either plain or in 8.25% dextrose. My impression is that the clinical difference between 0.5% tetracaine and 0.75% bupivacaine as hyperbaric solutions is minimal. Bupivacaine is appropriate for procedures lasting up to 2 to 2.5 hours.

In addition to hyperbaric technique, local anesthetics can be mixed to produce hypobaric spinal anesthesia. The most common method of formulating a hypobaric solution is to mix tetracaine in a 0.1% to 0.33% solution with sterile water. It has also become evident that lidocaine can be mixed to provide useful hypobaric spinal anesthesia. This drug is diluted from a 2% solution with sterile water to make a 0.5% solution, a total of 30 to 40 mg utilized.

Many anesthesiologists avoid vasoconstrictors for fear that their use somehow increases the risk in spinal anesthesia. These anesthesiologists believe that phenylephrine or epinephrine has such potent vasconstrictive action that it puts the blood supply of the spinal cord at risk. There are no human data supporting this theory. In fact, since most local anesthetics are vasodilators, the addition of these vasoconstrictors does little more than maintain spinal cord blood flow at a basal level. Commonly used doses for these vasoconstrictors are 0.2 mg of epinephrine and 5 mg of phenylephrine added to the spinal anesthetic.

Placement

Anatomy. A concept important to lumbar spinal anesthesia is illustrated in Figure 38–1. As outlined in Chapter 37, Centroneuraxis Anatomy, spinous processes of the lumbar vertebrae have an almost horizontal relationship to the long axis of their respective

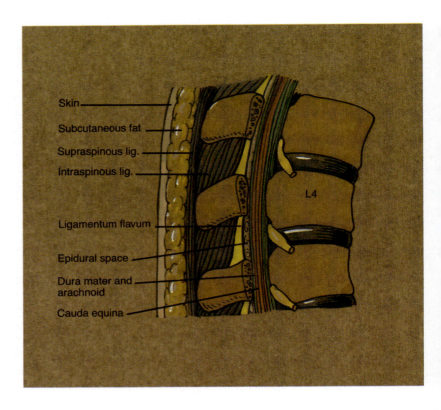

Skin
Subcutaneous fat
Supraspinous lig.
Intraspinous lig.

Ligamentum flavum

Epidural space

Dura mater and arachnoid

Cauda equina

L4

Figure 38—1 Spinal block—functional lumbar anatomy

vertebral bodies. When a midline needle is inserted between lumbar vertebral spines, it is most effective if it is placed in an almost perpendicular relationship to the long axis of the back. To facilitate spinal anesthesia, the anesthesiologist must constantly keep in mind the midline of the patient's body and centroneuraxis in relationship to the needle. As illustrated in Figure 38—1, from the surface inward as the midline needle is placed into the cerebrospinal fluid (CSF), it logically must puncture skin, subcutaneous tissue, superspinous ligament, interspinous ligament, ligamentum flavum, epidural space, and finally the dura and arachnoid mater to reach the CSF.

Position. Spinal anesthesia is carried out in three principal positions: lateral decubitus (Fig. 38—2), sitting (Fig. 38—3A and B), and prone jackknife (Fig. 38—4). In both the lateral decubitus and sitting positions, use of a well-trained assistant is essential if the block is to be easily administered by the anesthesiologist in a time-efficient manner. As illustrated in Figure 38—2, the assistant can help the patient assume the position of legs flexed upon the abdomen and chin flexed upon the chest. This is most easily accomplished by having the assistant pull the head toward the

chest, place an arm behind the patient's knees, and "push" the head and knees together. The position can also be facilitated by using an appropriate amount of sedation that allows the patient to be relaxed yet cooperative.

In some patients, the sitting position can facilitate location of the midline, especially in obese patients or in those with some scoliosis that makes midline identification more difficult. As illustrated in Figure 38—3A, the patient should assume a comfortable sitting position, with legs placed over the edge of the operating table and feet supported by a stool. A pillow should be placed in the patient's lap and the patient's arms allowed to drape over the pillow, resting on the flexed lower extremities. The assistant should be positioned immediately in front of the patient, supporting the shoulders and allowing the patient to minimize lumbar lordosis, while ensuring that the vertebral midline remains in a vertical position (Fig. 38—3B).

Sometimes it is more time-efficient to place the patient in a prone jackknife position prior to administration of the spinal anesthetic (Fig. 38—4). An assistant is not as essential for this technique as with the lateral decubitus and sitting positions, although, to

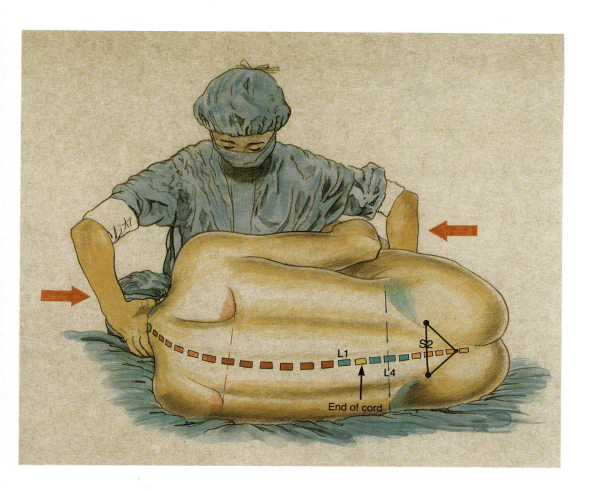

Figure 38–2 Spinal block—lateral decubitus position

Figure 38–3 Spinal block—sitting position—*A,* lateral view

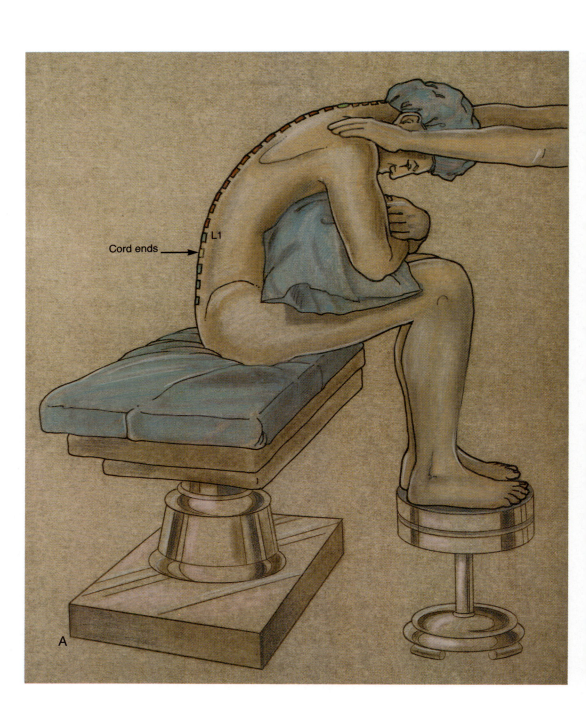

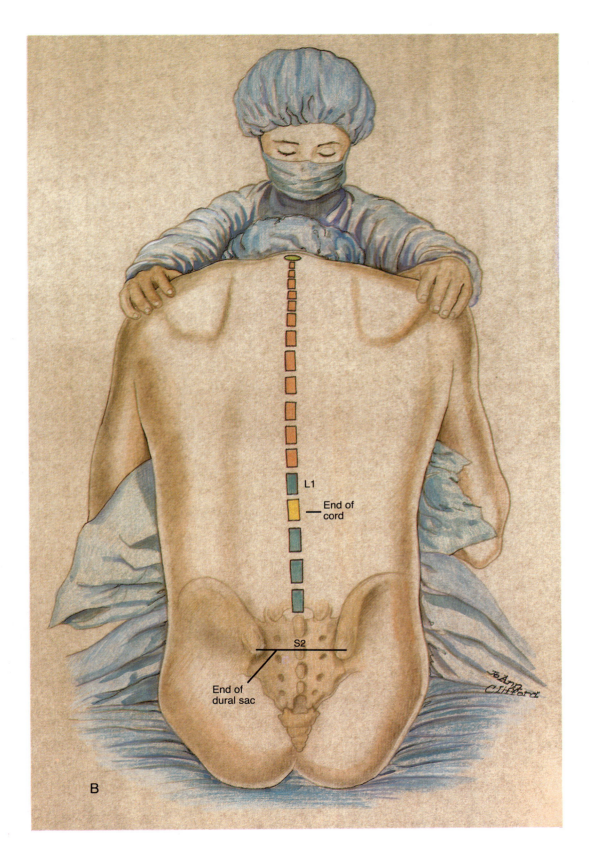

Figure 38–3 *continued* *B*, Posterior view

Figure 38–4 Spinal block—prone jack-knife position

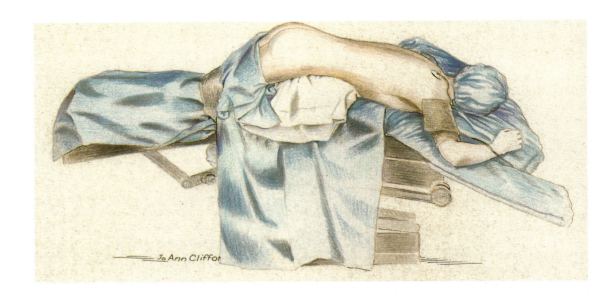

Figure 38–5 Spinal block—lumbar vertebra—lumbar lordosis present—inadequate positioning

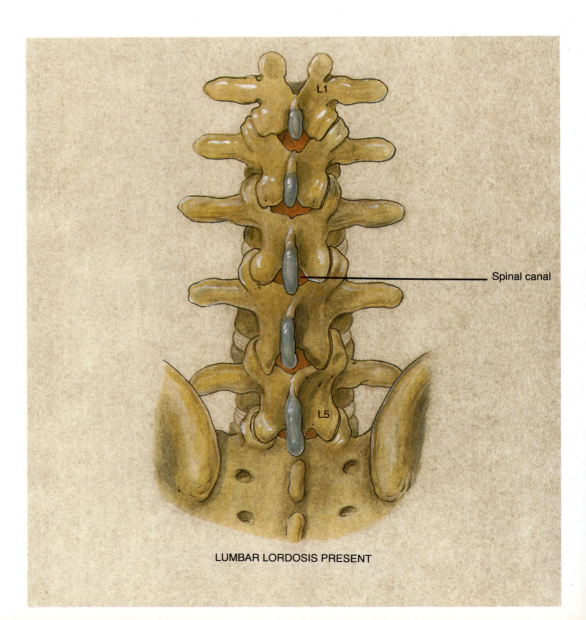

LUMBAR LORDOSIS PRESENT

make operating room block time efficient, it is often helpful if the assistant positions the patient in the prone jackknife position while the anesthesiologist readies the spinal anesthesia tray and drugs.

In all three positions, the goal is to so place the patient that the midline is readily identifiable and lumbar lordosis has been reduced. Figure 38–5 shows what the lumbar anatomy looks like when the patient's lumbar lordosis has been ineffectively reduced by poor positioning. As illustrated, the intralaminal space is small and difficult to enter with a needle in the midline. In contrast, Figure 38–6 illustrates how effective positioning can open the intralaminal space to allow easy access for subarachnoid puncture.

Needle Puncture. One of the first decisions in considering spinal anesthesia is what kind of needle to use. Although there are many eponyms for spinal needles, they fall into two main categories: those that cut the dura and those designed to spread dural fibers. The former include the traditional disposable spinal needle, the Quincke-Babcock needle, and the latter category contain the Greene needle. If a continuous spinal technique is chosen, the use of a Tuohy or other thin-walled needle will facilitate passage of the catheter. To make a logical choice of spinal

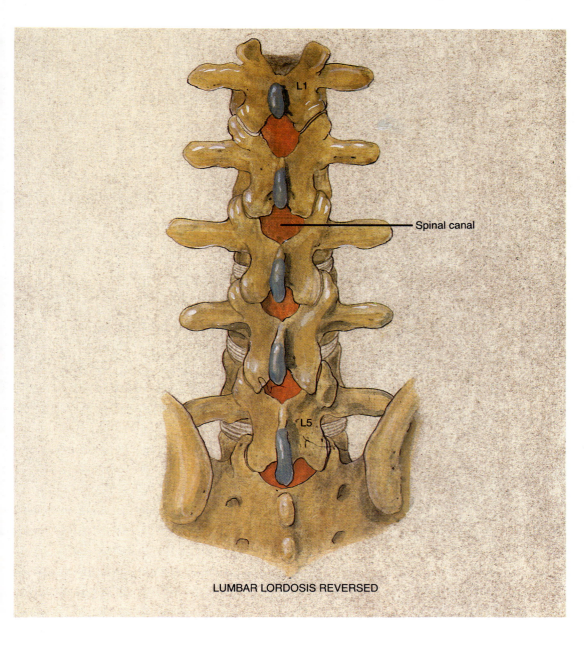

Figure 38–6 Spinal block—lumbar vertebra—lumbar lordosis reversed—ideal spinal positioning

Spinal canal

LUMBAR LORDOSIS REVERSED

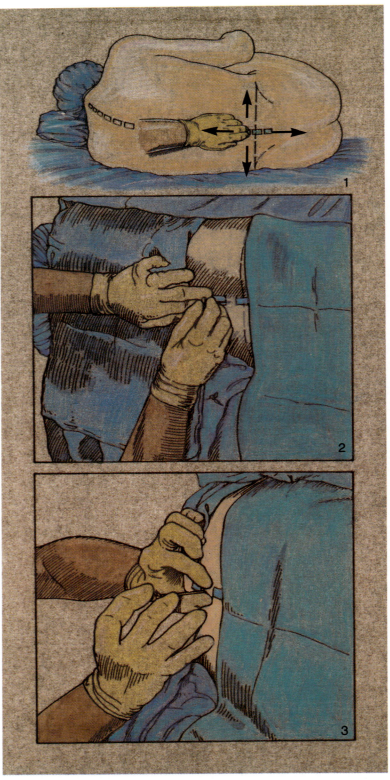

Figure 38—7 Spinal
block—technique

needle, the risks and benefits of each must be understood. The use of small needles reduces the incidence of postdural puncture headache; the use of larger needles improves the tactile "sense" of needle placement, thus increasing operator confidence.

It is probable that the risk-benefit equation is not as simple as this. For example, the use of a small needle, such as a 26-gauge needle, will not decrease headache incidence in younger patients if a number of "passes" through the dura are required until CSF flow is recognized. Likewise, a larger needle, such as a 22-gauge Greene, may result in a lower postdural puncture headache incidence if subarachnoid needle location is recognized on the first pass. Different needle tip designs may cause a difference in postdural puncture headache incidence, even when needle sizes are comparable.

With the patient in the proper position, the anesthesiologist uses the palpating hand to identify clearly the patient's intervertebral space and midline. As illustrated in Figure 38—7, the palpating hand can effectively carry out this important locating maneuver by moving the fingers in an alternating cephalocaudal direction, as well as rolling them from side to side. When the appropriate intervertebral space has been clearly identified, a skin wheal is raised over the space. Next, an introducer is inserted into the substance of the interspinous ligament, taking care to firmly seat it midline (Fig. 38—7, Step 2). Then the introducer is grasped with the palpating fingers and steadied while the other hand holds the spinal needle, somewhat like a dart, as illustrated in Figure 38—7, Step 3. With the fifth finger of the needle hand used as a tripod against the patient's back, the needle, with bevel (if present) parallel to the longitudinal dural fibers, is advanced slowly, to heighten the sense of tissue planes traversed, as well as to avoid skewing nerve roots, until a characteristic change in resistance is noted as the needle passes through ligamentum flavum and dura. The stylet is then removed, and CSF should appear at the needle hub. If it does not, the needle is rotated in 90° increments until CSF appears. If CSF does not appear in any quadrant, the needle should be advanced a few millimeters and rechecked in all four quadrants. If CSF still has not appeared and the needle is at a depth appropriate for the patient, the needle and introducer should be withdrawn and the insertion steps repeated, for the most common reason for lack of CSF return is the needle being inserted off the midline. Another common error preventing subarachnoid placement is for the anesthesiologist to insert the needle with too great a cephalic angle on the initial needle insertion (Fig. 38–8).

Once CSF is freely obtained, the dorsum of the anesthesiologist's nondominant hand steadies the spinal needle against the patient's back while the syringe containing the therapeutic dose is attached to the needle. CSF is again freely aspirated into the syringe and the dose injected. Sometimes, when the syringe has been attached to a needle from which CSF was clearly previously dripping, aspiration of additional CSF is impossible. As illustrated in Figure 38–9, one technique that can be utilized to help facilitate CSF aspiration is to "unscrew" the syringe plunger rather than provide constant steady pressure as an aid.

After the local anesthetic has been injected, the patient and operating table should be placed in the position appropriate for the surgical procedure and drugs chosen. The midline approach to subarachnoid block is the technique of first choice, since it requires anatomic projection in only two planes, and the plane is a relatively avascular one. When difficulties with needle insertion are encountered with the midline approach, an option is to use the paramedian route, which does not require the same level of patient cooperation or reversal of lumbar lordosis to be successful. As illustrated in Fig. 38–10, the paramedian approach exploits the larger "subarachnoid target" that exists if a needle is inserted slightly lateral to the midline. In the paramedian approach, the palpating fingers should identify the caudal edge of the cephalic spinous process of the intervertebral space chosen, and a skin wheal should be raised 1 cm lateral and 1 cm caudal to this point. A longer needle, such as a 4-cm, 22-gauge, short-beveled needle, is then used to infiltrate deeper tissues in a cephalomedial plane. The spinal introducer and needle are then inserted 10° to 15° off the sagittal plane in a cephalomedial plane, as noted in Figure 38–10. As with the midline approach, the most common error made with this tech-

Figure 38–8 Spinal block—avoiding too large a cephalic angle on insertion

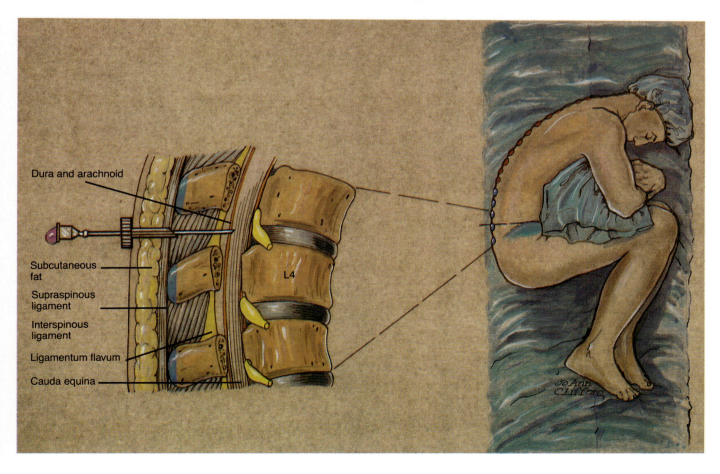

Dura and arachnoid

Subcutaneous fat

Supraspinous ligament

Interspinous ligament

Ligamentum flavum

Cauda equina

L4

Figure 38–9 Spinal block—syringe technique—facilitating cerebrospinal fluid aspiration

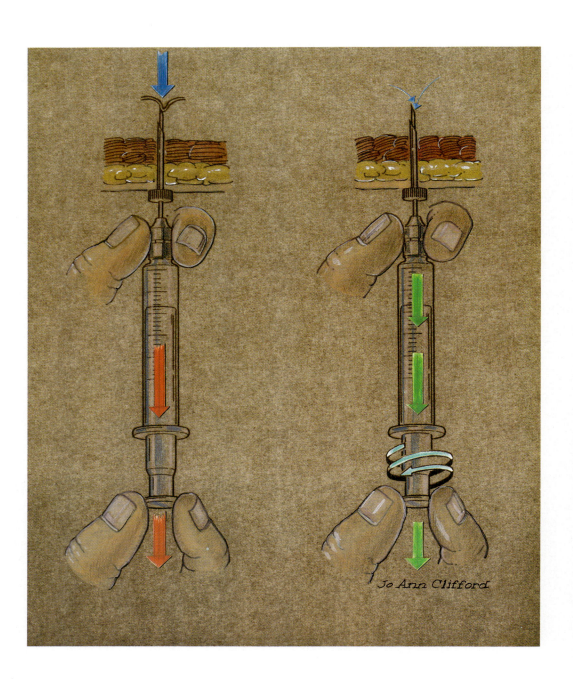

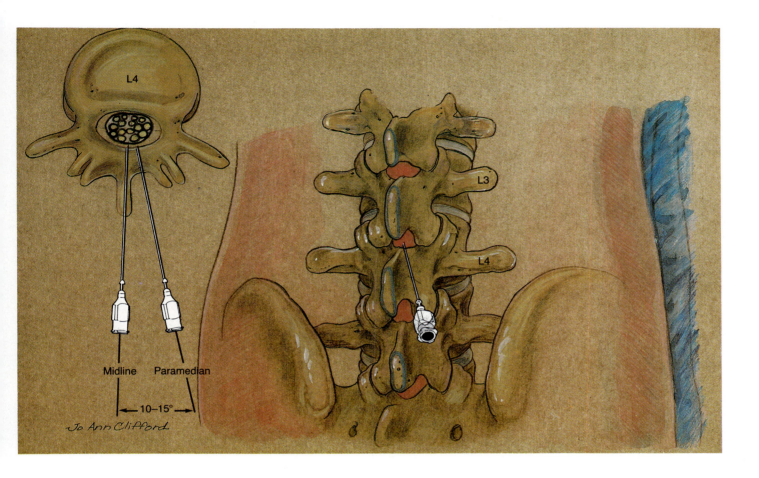

Figure 38—10 Spinal block—paramedian technique

nique is to angle the needle too far cephalad on the initial insertion of the needle. Once the needle contacts bone with this approach, it is redirected slightly in a cephalic direction. If bone is again contacted after needle redirection, but at a deeper level, this needle redirection is continued since it is likely that the needle is being "walked up" the lamina toward the intervertebral space. After CSF is obtained, the block is similar to that described for the midline approach.

A variation of the paramedian approach is the lumbosacral approach of Taylor. The technique is carried out at the L5/S1 interspace, the largest interlaminal interspace of the vertebral column. As illustrated in Figure 38—11, the skin insertion site is 1 cm medial and 1 cm caudal to the ipsilateral posterosuperior iliac spine. Through this point, a 12- to 15-cm spinal needle is inserted in a cephalomedial direction toward the midline. If

bone is encountered on the first needle insertion, the needle is walked off the sacrum into the subarachnoid space, similar to the method for a lumbar paramedian approach. Once CSF is obtained, the steps are similar to those previously outlined.

Potential Problems. The complication most feared by patients and many anesthesiologists after spinal anesthesia is neurologic injury. Admittedly, neurologic injury can occur after spinal anesthesia; however, to use spinal anesthesia appropriately, the risk-benefit equation of overall anesthesia neurologic injury must include those cases of neurologic injury that are possible following general anesthesia. If these comparisons are made, it is likely that neurologic injury following spinal anesthesia is in fact lower than that following general anesthesia. However, this must remain speculative.

Additionally, in those patients in whom

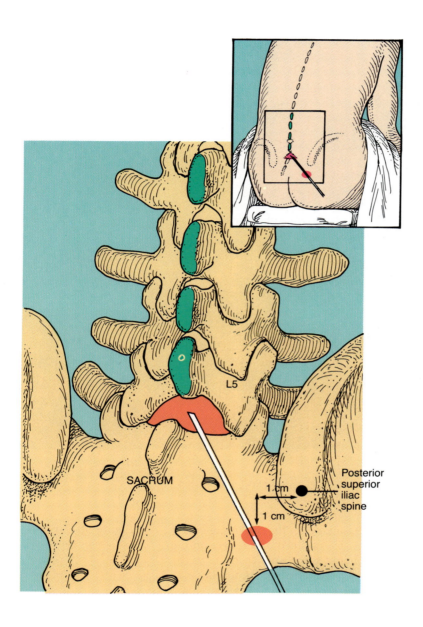

A more common complication of spinal anesthesia is postoperative headache. Factors that influence the incidence of postdural headache are age (more frequent in younger patients), gender (female patients more likely than male patients), needle size (more frequent with larger needles), needle bevel orientation (increased incidence when dural fibers are cut transversely), pregnancy (incidence increased), and number of dural punctures necessary to obtain CSF (more with multiple punctures). Perhaps more important than knowing the variables resulting in an increased incidence of postdural puncture headache is the knowledge of how and when to carry out definitive therapy—that is, epidural blood patch. To use spinal anesthesia effectively, epidural blood patching, when indicated, must be used early. The success rate from a single epidural blood patch should be in the 90% to 95% range, and, if a second patch is required, a similar percentage should be obtainable.

One other common side effect of spinal anesthesia is that approximately 25% of patients will have a backache following the procedure. Patients often blame "the spinal" for backache; but, when looked at systematically, it appears that as many patients have backache following general anesthesia as following spinal anesthesia. Thus, backache after centroneuraxis block should not be attributed immediately to "needling" of the back.

Pearls

Probably the most important factor for success with spinal anesthesia in the day-to-day life of an anesthesiologist is that the technique must be time-efficient. Use of spinal anesthesia cannot measurably add to the surgical day if nurses and surgeons are to be co-advocates of this technique. Thus, one should plan ahead to maximize efficiency. Often overlooked in this maxim is that patient preparation for operation can begin almost as soon as the block is administered, if the patient is properly sedated.

Intraoperatively, during high spinal anesthesia (often during cesarean section) patients will occasionally complain excessively of dyspnea. This often appears to be

Figure 38–11 Spinal block—L5/S1 paramedian technique—Taylor's approach

the spinal block level needs to be precisely controlled, or in those patients with operations expected to outlast usual anesthetic drug durations, a continuous spinal catheter may be used. However, when using a continuous spinal technique be cautious about repeating local anesthetic injections if the block height does not reach predicted levels. It has been hypothesized that neurotoxicity (cauda equina syndrome) is possible when spinal catheter position allows local anesthetic concentrations to reach higher than expected levels.

a result of loss of chest wall sensation rather than of significantly decreased inspiratory capacity. The loss of chest wall sensation does not allow the patients to experience the reassurance of a deep breath. This impediment to patient acceptance often can be overcome simply by having patients raise a hand in front of the mouth and exhale forcefully. The tactile appreciation of a deep exhalation often seems to provide the needed reassurance.

If spinal anesthesia has been used and a neurologic complication is noted postoperatively, it is essential to obtain neurologic consultation early. In this way, an unbiased consultant can examine the patient and determine whether the "new" neurologic finding was preexistent, related to a peripheral neuropathy, or, more rarely, potentially related to the spinal anesthetic. The latency in electromyographic alterations associated with denervation due to neurologic injury takes time to develop in the lower extremities (14 to 21 days). Therefore, following a potentially spinal-related lesion, electromyographic studies should be obtained early and serially.

39

Epidural Block

Perspective

Epidural anesthesia is the second primary method of centroneuraxis block. In contrast to spinal anesthesia, epidural blockade requires pharmacologic doses of local anesthetics, making systemic toxicity a concern. In skilled hands, the incidence of postdural puncture headache should be lower with epidural anesthesia than with spinal anesthesia. Nevertheless, as outlined in Chapter 38, Spinal Block, I do not believe this should be the major differentiating point between the two techniques. Spinal anesthesia, typically, is a single-shot technique, whereas frequently intermittent injection is done through an epidural catheter, thus allowing reinjection and prolongation of epidural blockade. Another difference is that epidural blockade allows production of segmental anesthesia. Thus, if a thoracic injection is made and an appropriate amount of local anesthetic injected, a band of anesthesia can be produced that does not block the lower extremities.

Patient Selection. Epidural blockade is appropriate for virtually the same patients as is spinal anesthesia, with the exception that epidural anesthesia can be used in the cervical and thoracic areas—levels at which spinal anesthesia is not advised. As with spinal anesthesia, if epidural blockade is to be used for intra-abdominal procedures involving the upper abdomen, it is advisable to combine the technique with a light general anesthetic, since diaphragmatic irritation can make the patient, surgeon, and anesthesiologist uncomfortable. Other patients for epidural anesthesia are those in whom a continuous technique has been found increasingly helpful in providing epidural local anesthetic and/or opioid analgesia postoperatively following major surgical procedures. This application alone probably explains the increased interest in epidural block.

Pharmacologic Choice. To utilize epidural local anesthetics effectively, one must combine an understanding of local anesthetic potency and duration with estimates of length of the operation and postoperative analgesia requirements. Drugs available for epidural use can be categorized into short, intermediate, and long-acting agents; with the addition of epinephrine to these agents, surgical anesthesia ranging from 45 to 240 minutes is possible.

Chloroprocaine, an amino ester local anesthetic, is a short-acting agent that allows an efficient matching of surgical procedure length and duration of epidural analgesia, even in outpatients. 2-Chloroprocaine is available in 2% and 3% concentrations, with the latter preferable for surgical anesthesia and the former for techniques not requiring muscle relaxation.

Lidocaine is the prototypical amino amide local anesthetic and is used in 1.5% and 2% concentrations epidurally. Mepivacaine concentrations necessary for epidural anesthesia are similar to those of lidocaine; however, mepivacaine lasts from 15 to 30 minutes longer at equivalent dosages. Epinephrine significantly prolongs the duration of surgical anesthesia with 2-chloroprocaine and both lidocaine and mepivacaine—i.e., approximately 50%. Plain lidocaine will produce surgical anesthesia lasting from 60 to 100 minutes.

Bupivacaine, an amino amide, is the most widely used long-acting local anesthetic for epidural anesthesia, and it is used in 0.5% and 0.75% concentrations. Analgesic techniques can be performed with concentrations of from 0.125% to 0.25%. Its duration of action is not as consistently prolonged by the addition of epinephrine, although up to 240 minutes of surgical anesthesia can be obtained when epinephrine is added.

In addition to epinephrine as an additive, some anesthetists recommend modifying epidural local anesthetic solutions as a means of increasing both speed of onset and quality of the block produced. One recommendation is to carbonate the local anesthetic solution. I believe this unnecessarily complicates clinical epidural anesthesia and as yet shows no clear clinical advantage. The addition of bicarbonate also has been suggested as a means of increasing the speed of onset, as well as prolonging the block. Despite statistically significant increases in speed of onset, the clinical significance of adding bicarbonate to local anesthetic solution, again, awaits larger studies showing clinical utility.

Placement

Anatomy. As with spinal anesthesia, the key to carrying out successful epidural anesthesia is an understanding of midline centroneuraxis anatomy. As illustrated in Figure

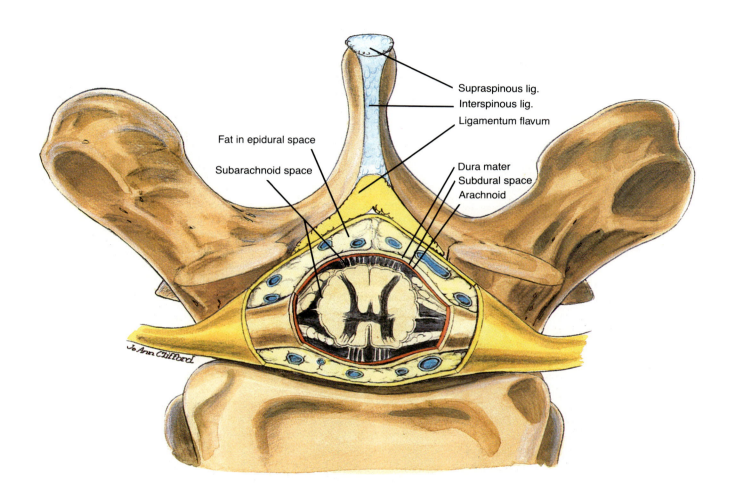

Supraspinous lig.
Interspinous lig.
Ligamentum flavum

Fat in epidural space

Subarachnoid space

Dura mater
Subdural space
Arachnoid

Jo Ann Clifford

Figure 39—1 Epidural block—cross-sectional anatomy

39—1, it is essential for the anesthesiologist to create a "3-D" image of the centroneuraxis midline structures that underlie palpating fingers. When a lumbar approach to the epidural space is used, the depth from the skin to the ligamentum flavum commonly approaches 4 cm; 80% of patients have an epidural space cannulated at between 3.5 and 6 cm from the skin. In this lumbar region, the ligamentum flavum is 5 to 6 mm thick in the midline, whereas in the thoracic region it is from 3 to 5 mm thick. It is emphasized that if needles are kept in the midline, the ligamentum flavum will be perceived as a thicker ligament than if needles are allowed to be inserted off the midline and entered at the

lateral extension of the ligamentum flavum. Figure 39—2 illustrates how important it is to maintain midline position of the epidural needle. If an oblique approach is taken, a "false release" can be produced (*needle C*), or the perception of a "thin" ligament reinforced (*needle B*).

Position. Positioning for epidural anesthesia is similar to that for spinal anesthesia, with lateral decubitus, sitting, and prone jackknife positions all applicable. The lateral decubitus position is applicable to both lumbar and thoracic epidural anesthesia, and the sitting position allows both lumbar and thoracic as well as cervical epidural anesthesia to be administered. The prone jackknife posi-

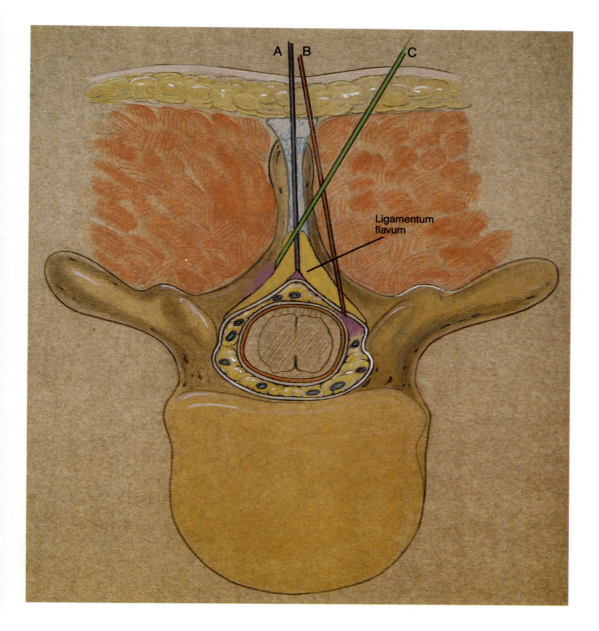

Ligamentum
flavum

Figure 39–2 Epidural block—functional ligamentum flavum anatomy

tion allows access to the caudal epidural space.

Needle Puncture. A technique similar to that used for spinal anesthesia should be carried out to identify midline structures, while bony landmarks should be utilized to determine the vertebral level appropriate for needle insertion (Fig. 39–3). When choosing a needle for epidural anesthesia, a decision must be made about a continuous or single-shot technique. This is the principal determi-

nant of needle selection. If a single-shot epidural technique is chosen, a Crawford needle is appropriate; if a continuous catheter technique is indicated, either a Tuohy or other needle with lateral facing opening is chosen.

If a lumbar epidural anesthetic is to be carried out, the midline approach is most often indicated. The needle is inserted into the midline in the same way as that for spinal anesthesia. With the epidural technique, the needle is slowly advanced until the change in

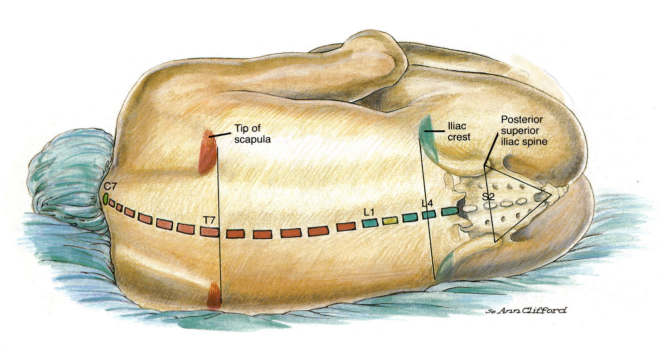

Figure 39—3 Centroneuraxis anatomy—surface relationships

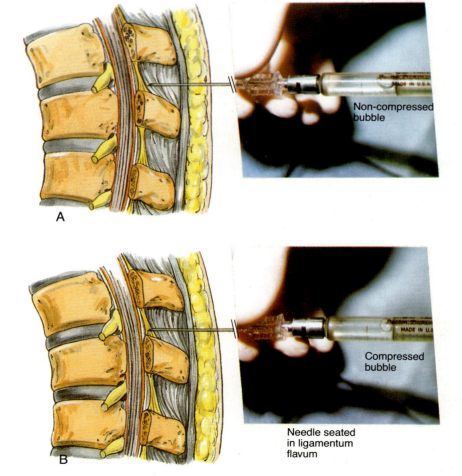

Figure 39—4 Epidural block—loss of resistance technique—bubble compression

tissue resistance is noted as the needle abuts the ligamentum flavum. At this point, a 3- to 5-ml glass syringe is filled with 2 ml of saline and a small (0.25 ml) air bubble is added. As illustrated in Figure 39–4, the syringe is attached to the needle and, if the needle tip is in the substance of the ligamentum flavum, the air bubble will be compressible, as illustrated in Figure 39–4B. If the ligamentum flavum has not yet been reached, pressure on the syringe plunger will not compress the air bubble (Fig. 39–4A). Once compression of the air bubble has been achieved, the needle is grasped with the nondominant hand and pulled toward the epidural space, while the dominant hand (thumb) applies constant, steady pressure on the syringe plunger, thus compressing the air bubble. When the epidural space is entered, the pressure applied to the syringe plunger will allow the solution to flow without resistance into the epidural space.

An alternative technique, though with a less precise endpoint, I believe, is the hanging-drop identification of entry into the epidural space. In this technique, when the needle is placed into the ligamentum flavum a drop of solution is placed within the hub of the needle. No syringe is attached and, when the needle is advanced into the epidural

space, the solution should be "sucked in" (Fig. 39–5).

No matter what method is chosen for needle insertion, when the epidural space is cannulated with a catheter, success may be increased by advancing the needle 1 to 2 mm more once the space is identified. Additionally, the incidence of unintentional intravenous cannulation with an epidural catheter may be lessened by injecting 5 to 10 ml of solution prior to threading the catheter. If a catheter is inserted, it should be inserted only 2 to 3 cm into the epidural space, since threading more of the catheter may increase the likelihood of catheter malposition.

Potential Problems. One of the most feared complications of epidural anesthesia is systemic toxicity resulting from intravenous injection of the intended epidural anesthetic dose (Fig. 39–6). This can occur with either catheter or needle injections. One way to avoid intravenous injection of the pharmacologic doses of local anesthetic needed for epidural anesthesia is to administer a test dose prior to epidural injection. Currently the recommendation is to use 3 ml of local anesthetic solution containing 1:200,000 epinephrine (15 µg of epinephrine). In spite of a negative test dose, anesthesiologists should inject incrementally, be vigilant for uninten-

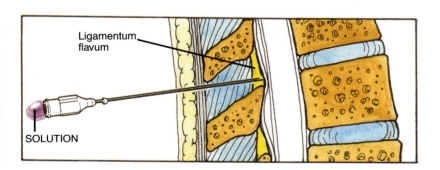

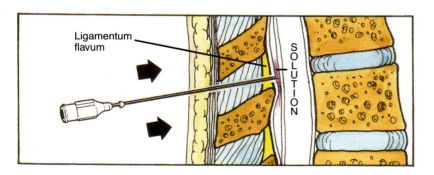

Figure 39–5 Epidural block—hanging drop technique

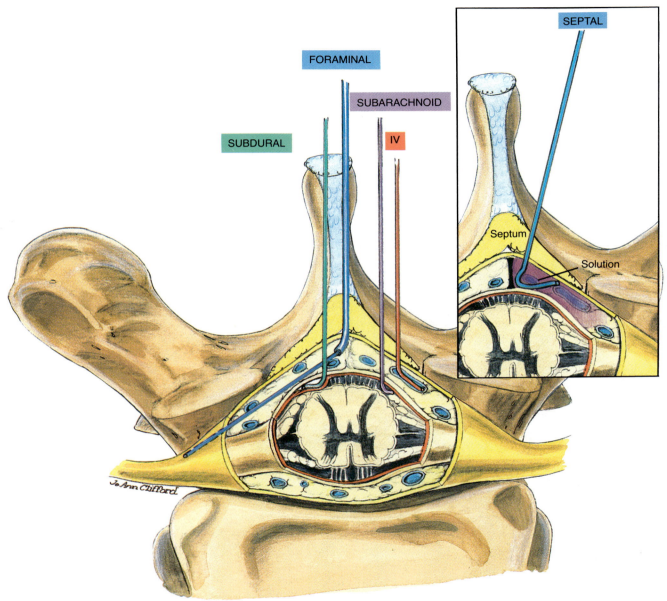

Figure 39–6 Epidural block—cross-sectional anatomy—potential complications

tional intravascular injection, and have all necessary equipment and drugs available to treat local anesthetic-induced systemic toxicity.

Another problem that can occur with epidural injection is the unintentional administration of an epidural dose into the spinal fluid. As with any centroneuraxis block that reaches high sensory levels, blood pressure and heart rate should be supported pharmacologically and ventilation assisted as indicated. Usually atropine and ephedrine will suffice or at least provide one the time to administer more potent catecholamines. If the entire dose (20 to 25 ml) of local anesthetic was administered into the CSF, tracheal intu-

bation and mechanical ventilation are indicated since it will be approximately 1 to 2 hours until the patient will consistently maintain adequate spontaneous ventilation after such an event. When an epidural anesthetic is performed and a higher than expected block develops only after a delay of 15 to 30 minutes, subdural placement of the local anesthetic must be considered. Treatment is symptomatic, with the most difficult part of treatment involving the recognition that a subdural injection is possible.

As with spinal anesthesia, if neurologic injury occurs following epidural technique, a systematic approach to the problem needs to be carried out. No particular local anesthetic, needle vs. catheter technique, addition or omission of epinephrine, or location of epidural puncture seems associated with an increased incidence of neurologic injury.

An additional problem with epidural anesthesia is the fear that an epidural hematoma will be created with the epidural needles or catheters. This is probably of less frequency than severe neurologic injury following general anesthesia. Concern over epidural hematoma formation is increased in patients who have been taking antiplatelet drugs, such as aspirin, or who have been receiving anticoagulants preoperatively. The acceptable magnitude of preoperative anticoagulation and risk-benefit of performing epidural anesthesia must remain indeterminate at this time. The use of epidural techniques in patients receiving subcutaneous heparin therapy is probably acceptable if the block can be performed atraumatically, though the risk-benefit of the technique must be weighed for each patient.

As in spinal anesthesia, postdural puncture headache can result from epidural anesthesia when unintentional subarachnoid puncture accompanies the technique. When using the larger diameter epidural needles (18- and 19-gauge), it can be expected that at least 50% of patients experiencing an unintentional dural puncture will have a headache postoperatively.

Pearls

If catheters can be avoided during epidural anesthesia—that is, by selecting an appropriate local anesthetic, a potential source of difficulties with the technique can also be avoided. There are a number of ways epidural catheters can be malpositioned. If catheters are inserted too far into the epidural space, they can be routed out the foramina and result in patchy epidural blockade. The catheter can also be inserted into the subdural or subarachnoid space, or into an epidural vein. Similarly, epidural catheter use may be complicated by a prominent dorsomedian connective tissue band (epidural septum) found in some patients.

Another means of facilitating successful use of epidural anesthesia is to allow the block enough "soak time" prior to the surgical procedure. This is most effectively accomplished if the block is carried out in an induction room separate from the operating room. Be aware that there appears to be a plateau effect in dosing epidural local anesthetics. That is, once some quantity of local anesthetic has been injected, more local anesthetic does not significantly increase the block height but rather may make the block denser—perhaps improving quality.

One observation about epidural anesthesia via a catheter that needs reemphasis is the often faulty "clinical logic" that, by giving incremental doses through a catheter, the level of sensory anesthesia can be slowly developed, thereby allowing frail and physiologically compromised patients to undergo epidural anesthesia. I believe often the logic behind this concept is flawed. Usually when this approach is taken, anesthesiologists do not allow enough time between injections because of the reality of time pressures in the normal operating room. They inject small doses through the catheter, then do not allow sufficient time to pass before the next incremental injection. Often the clinical result is high block levels in just those patients in whom lower levels were the goal. Furthermore, this approach to epidural anesthesia unnecessarily delays making the patient ready for operation and makes surgical and nursing colleagues less accepting of the technique.

Epidural catheters are indicated in some situations, especially when the technique is used for postoperative analgesia. In order to place a known length of catheter into the epidural space, the catheter has to be marked and either a way found to maintain catheter position once the needle is withdrawn over the catheter, or else both the needle and catheter must have distance markings. Many epidural needles do not have distance markers, so that a method is required of maintaining catheter position while the needle is withdrawn over the catheter. One technique of catheter positioning is illustrated in Figure 39–7. Select an object of known length, such as a syringe or the anesthesiologist's finger, and place that object next to the

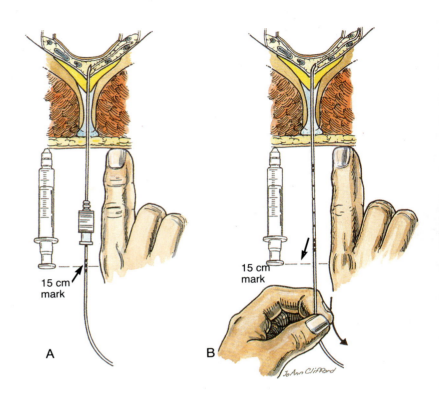

Figure 39—7 Epidural block—catheter measurement technique

A

B

needle catheter assembly after the catheter has been placed 3 cm into the epidural space. Since the catheter is marked, some known point on the catheter can be conceptually related to a known point on either the finger or syringe. As shown in Figure 39—7A, the 15-cm mark is opposite the plunger on the syringe, or the anesthesiologist's knuckle. Once this relationship has been noted, the needle is removed while the catheter position is maintained. The measurement object is

then placed next to the catheter, as illustrated in Figure 39—7B, and the catheter is withdrawn to the point at which the distance marker on the catheter relates to the previously identified point. In this example, the 15-cm mark on the catheter is placed opposite the plunger of the syringe or the anesthesiologist's knuckle. By using this technique, the epidural catheter can be accurately placed without having either a marked needle or ruler.

40

Caudal Block

Perspective

Advances in lumbar epidural anesthesia have helped caudal anesthesia become an infrequently utilized and taught technique. Nevertheless, caudal anesthesia can be effectively used for anorectal and perineal procedures, as well as some lower extremity operations.

Patient Selection. Patient selection for caudal anesthesia should be determined realistically by anatomy of the sacral hiatus. In approximately 5% of patients the sacral hiatus will be nearly impossible to cannulate with needle or catheter, and thus in 1 of 20 patients the technique is clinically unusable. Likewise, there will be patients in whom tissue mass overlying the sacrum makes the technique difficult, and if another technique is applicable, caudal anesthesia should be avoided. Probably more so than for any other block, anesthesiologist experience and confidence with the technique are necessary in order to carry it out effectively.

Pharmacologic Choice. When choosing local anesthetics for caudal anesthesia, the same considerations as those for epidural anesthe-

sia are needed. It must be recognized that volumes of local anesthetic in the 25- to 35-ml range are necessary to predictably provide a sensory level of T12 to T10 with caudal injection.

Placement

Anatomy. Anatomy pertinent to caudal anesthesia centers upon the sacral hiatus (Fig. 40–1). This can be most effectively localized by finding the posterosuperior iliac spines bilaterally, drawing a line to join them, and then completing an equilateral triangle in a caudal direction. The tip of the equilateral triangle will overlie the sacral hiatus (Fig. 40–2). The caudal tip of the triangle will rest near the sacral cornua, which are unfused remnants of the spinous processes of the fifth sacral vertebra. Overlying the sacral hiatus is a fibroelastic membrane, which is the functional counterpart of the ligamentum flavum. Perhaps more than with any other gender difference in regional anesthesia, the sacrum is distinctly different between male and female. In men, the cavity of the sacrum

Figure 40–1 Caudal block—surface anatomy

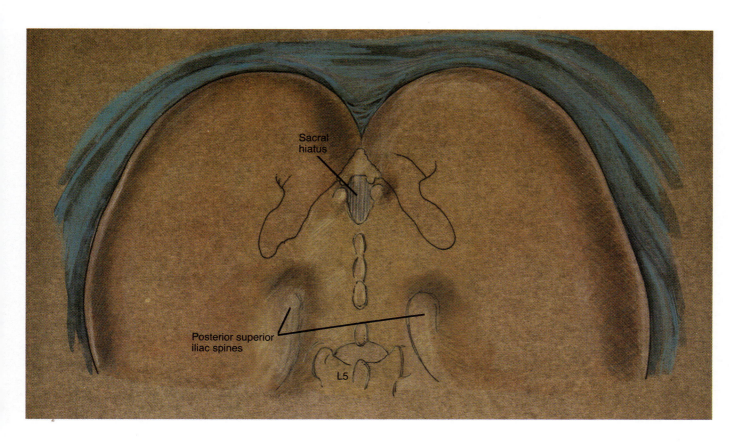

Sacral
hiatus

Posterior superior
iliac spines

L5

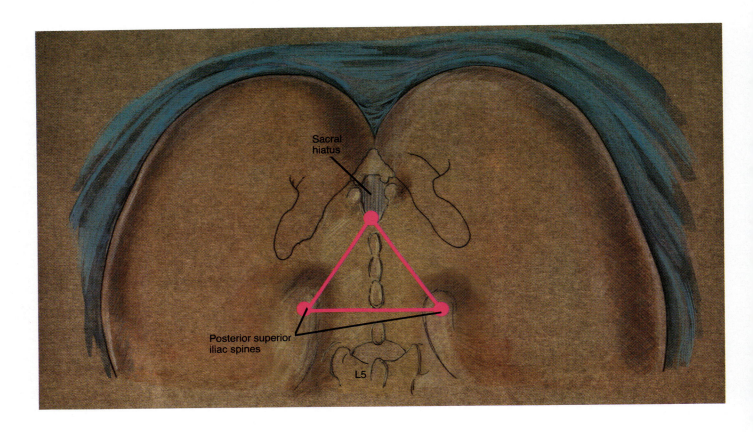

Sacral
hiatus

Posterior superior
iliac spines

L5

Figure 40–2 Caudal block—surface anatomy—sacral hiatus localization

has a smooth curve from S1 to S5. Conversely, in women, the sacrum is quite flat from S1 to S3, with a more pronounced curve in the S4/S5 region (Fig. 40–3).

Position. Caudal blockade can be carried out in a lateral decubitus position or a prone position. In adults, I find the prone position with a pillow placed beneath the lower abdomen most effective. In this position, patients can be sufficiently sedated to make the block comfortable, and for me it makes the midline more easily identifiable than in the lateral position. As illustrated in Figure 40–4, pediatric caudal anesthesia is commonly carried out with the child in the lateral decubitus position. Since most pediatric caudal blocks are performed after induction with general anesthesia, the lateral position is almost mandatory. Identification of the midline and performance of the block are less complicated in the pediatric patient, thus making the lateral position clinically useful. To maximize identification of the sacral hiatus, the prone patient should have the legs abducted to a 20° angle and the toes rotated inward. This helps relax the gluteal muscles and al-

lows easier identification of the sacral hiatus (Fig. 40–5).

Needle Puncture. As with lumbar epidural anesthesia, caudal anesthesia requires a decision about the use of a single injection or a catheter technique. If a single-shot caudal anesthetic is to be performed, almost any needle of sufficient length to reach the caudal canal is applicable. In adults, a needle at least 22-gauge or larger is recommended, since it is large enough to allow sufficiently rapid injection of solution to help detect misplaced local anesthetic injections. If a catheter is to be utilized, a needle of sufficient size to allow catheter passage is required. As illustrated in Figure 40–6, after the sacral hiatus is identified, the index and middle fingers of the palpating hand are placed on the sacral cornu, and the caudal needle is inserted at an angle of approximately 45° to the sacrum. While the anesthesiologist advances the needle, a decrease in resistance to needle insertion should be appreciated as the needle enters the caudal canal. The needle is then advanced until bone is contacted; this should be the dorsal aspect of the ventral plate of

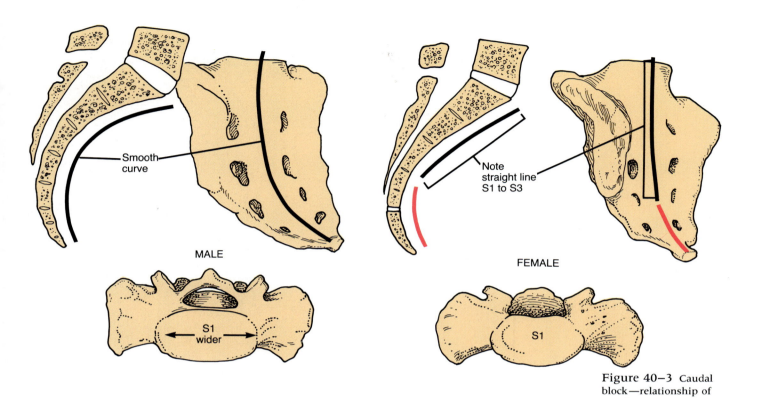

MALE

FEMALE

Smooth curve

Note straight line S1 to S3

S1 wider

S1

Figure 40–3 Caudal block—relationship of sacral anatomy to gender

Figure 40–4 Caudal block—pediatric position

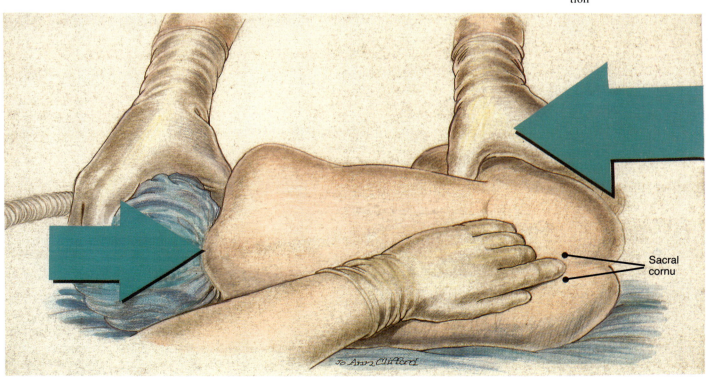

Sacral cornu

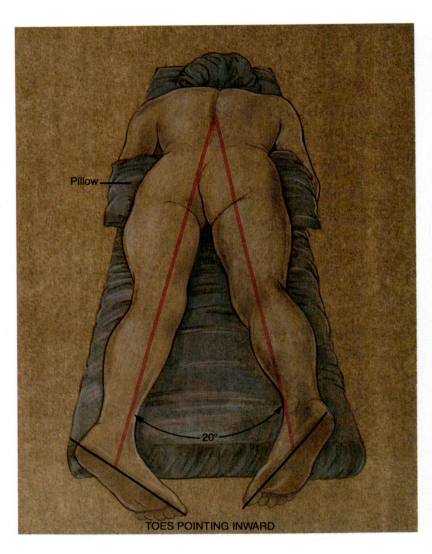

Pillow

20°

Figure 40—5 Caudal
block—prone position

TOES POINTING INWARD

the sacrum. The needle is then withdrawn slightly and redirected so that the angle of insertion relative to the skin surface is decreased. In male patients, this angle will be almost parallel to the tabletop, whereas in female patients a slightly steeper angle will be necessary.

During the redirection of the needle, and following loss of resistance, the needle should be advanced approximately 1 to 1.5 cm into the caudal canal. Further advance is not suggested, since dural puncture and unintentional intravascular cannulation become more likely. Prior to the injection of the therapeutic dose of local anesthetic, aspiration and a test dose should be carried out, since a vein or subarachnoid space can be entered unintentionally, as is the case in lumbar epidural anesthesia.

Potential Problems. Caudal anesthesia embodies most of the same complications that can accompany lumbar epidural anesthesia. One distinct difference, however, is that the incidence of subarachnoid puncture is exceedingly low with caudal technique. The dural sac ends at approximately the level of S2; thus, unless a needle is inserted deeply within the caudal canal, subarachnoid puncture is unlikely. It is emphasized that in children the dural sac is more distally placed in the caudal canal, and this should be considered when carrying out pediatric caudal anesthesia.

Perhaps the most frequent problem with caudal anesthesia is ineffective blockade, which results from a considerable variation in the anatomy of the sacral hiatus. If anesthesiologists are unfamiliar with caudal tech-

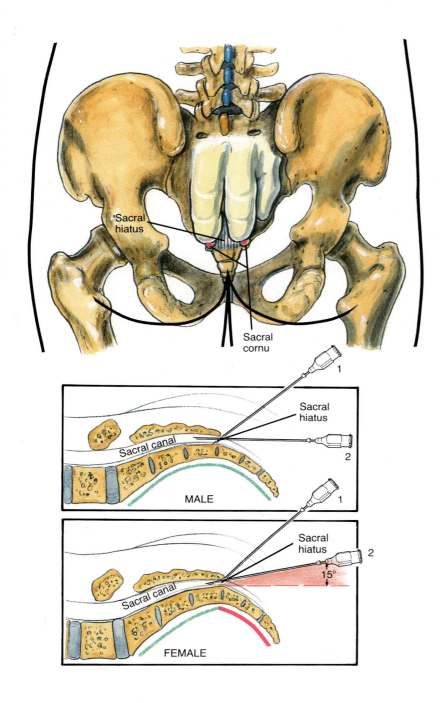

Figure 40−6 Caudal block—technique

nique and the needle passes anterior to the ventral plate of the sacrum, puncture of the rectum or, in the case of obstetric anesthesia, fetal parts, is possible. As illustrated in Fig. 40−7, the area surrounding the sacral hiatus can be imagined as a potential "circle of errors." You may be faced with a slitlike hiatus that does not allow easy needle insertion; the hiatus may be more cephalic than anticipated, or in fact be closed. Likewise, loss of resistance may be encountered as the needle is inserted into one of the sacral foramina rather than the hiatus. In the lateral view, it is obvious that needles may be misplaced in subcutaneous or periosteal locations, as well as into the marrow of sacral bones.

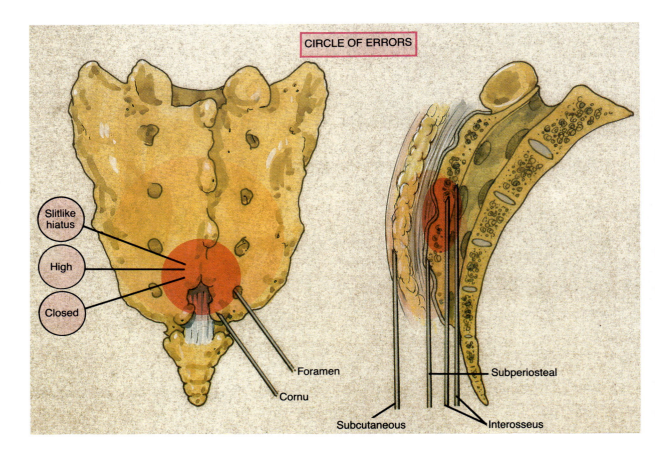

CIRCLE OF ERRORS

Slitlike hiatus

High

Closed

Foramen

Cornu

Subcutaneous

Subperiosteal

Interosseus

Figure 40–7 Caudal block—circle of errors

Pearls

To attain effective caudal anesthesia, anesthesiologists should be selective about the patients in whom it is attempted. It makes no sense to use the technique in a patient whose anatomy is unfavorable. Because of the anatomic variations surrounding the sacral hiatus, this block seems to require more operator experience and a longer time to proficiency than many other regional blocks. As a result, anesthesiologists should develop their technique on patients with favorable anatomy.

One helpful hint that will confirm needle location when carrying out caudal anesthesia is illustrated in Figure 40–8. Once the needle has entered what is thought to be the caudal canal, the anesthesiologist should place a palpating hand across the sacral region dorsally. Then 5 ml of saline should be rapidly injected through the caudal needle. By placing the hand as shown, the anesthesiologist should be immediately aware of subcutaneous needle positioning overlying the sacrum. If the needle is mispositioned subcutaneously, a "bulge" during injection will develop in the midline. If the needle is correctly positioned within the caudal canal, no midline bulge should be palpable. It is emphasized that, in thin individuals, accurate needle placement in the caudal canal and rapid injection of solution may allow the anesthesiologist to feel small pressure waves more laterally overlying the sacral foramina. Do not confuse these smaller pressure waves with those associated with a misplaced subcutaneous needle.

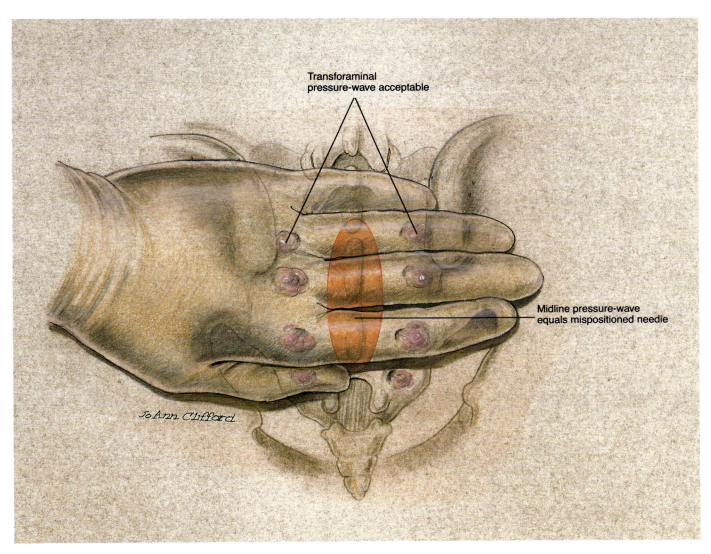

Transforaminal
pressure-wave acceptable

Midline pressure-wave
equals mispositioned needle

Jo Ann Clifford

Figure 40–8 Caudal
block—palpation
technique

References

General

Bonica JJ: The Management of Pain, Volumes I–II. 2nd ed. Lea & Febiger, Philadelphia, 1990.

Brown DL, Wedel DJ: Introduction to regional anesthesia. *In* Miller RD (ed): Anesthesia. 3rd ed. Churchill Livingstone, New York, 1990, pp 1369–1375.

Brown DL, Wedel DJ: Spinal, epidural and caudal anesthesia. *In* Miller RD (ed): Anesthesia. 3rd ed. Churchill Livingstone, New York, 1990, pp 1377–1405.

Brown DL (ed): Regional Anesthesia at Virginia Mason Medical Center: A Clinical Perspective. Problems in Anesthesia, Volume 1. JB Lippincott Company, Philadelphia, 1987.

Brown DL (ed): Perioperative Analgesia. Problems in Anesthesia, Volume 2. JB Lippincott Company, Philadelphia, 1988.

Carron H, Korbon GA, Rowlingson JC: Regional Anesthesia: Techniques and Clinical Applications. Grune & Stratton, Orlando, FL, 1984.

Christoforidis AJ: Atlas of Axial, Sagittal, and Coronal Anatomy, WB Saunders Company, Philadelphia, 1988.

Cousins M, Bridenbaugh PO (eds): Neural Blockade. 2nd ed. JB Lippincott Company, Philadelphia, 1988.

Covino BG, Scott DB: Handbook of Epidural Anaesthesia and Analgesia. Grune & Stratton, Orlando, FL, 1985.

Eriksson E (ed): Illustrated Handbook in Local Anaesthesia. 2nd ed. WB Saunders Company, Philadelphia, 1980.

Gosling JA, Harris PF, Humpherson JR, Whitmore I, Willan PLT: Atlas of Human Anatomy with Integrated Text. Gower Medical Publishing, London, 1985.

Grant JCB: An Atlas of Anatomy. 5th ed. Williams & Wilkins, Baltimore, 1962.

Katz J: Atlas of Regional Anesthesia. Appleton-Century-Crofts, Norwalk, CT, 1985.

Katz J, Renck H: Handbook of Thoraco-Abdominal Nerve Block. Grune & Stratton, Orlando, FL, 1987.

Labat G: Regional Anesthesia: Its Technique and Clinical Application, WB Saunders Company, Philadelphia, 1923.

McMinn RMH, Hutchings RT: Color Atlas of Human Anatomy. Year Book Medical Publishers, Chicago, 1977.

Melloni JL, Dox I, Melloni HP, Melloni BJ: Melloni's Illustrated Review of Human Anatomy. JB Lippincott Company, Philadelphia, 1988.

Moore DC: Regional Block. 4th ed., CC Thomas, Publisher, Springfield, IL, 1965.

Moore DC: Stellate Ganglion Block. CC Thomas, Publisher, Springfield, IL, 1954.

Raj PP: Handbook of Regional Anesthesia. Churchill Livingstone, New York, 1985.

Thompson GE, Brown DL: The common nerve blocks. *In* Nunn JF, Utting JE, Brown BR (eds): General Anaesthesia. 5th ed. Butterworth, London, 1989, pp 1049–1085.

Wedel DJ, Brown DL: Peripheral nerve blocks. *In* Miller RD (ed): Anesthesia. 3rd ed. Churchill Livingstone, New York, 1990, pp 1407–1437.

Winnie AP: Plexus Anesthesia, Volume I: Perivascular Techniques of Brachial Plexus Block. WB Saunders Company, Philadelphia, 1983.

Woodburne RT: Essentials of Human Anatomy. 5th ed. Oxford University Press, New York, 1973.

Introductory Chapter

Bashein G, Haschke RH, Ready LB: Electrical nerve location: Numerical and electrophoretic comparison of insulated vs uninsulated needles. Anesth Analg 63: 919–924, 1984.

Carpenter RL, Mackey DC: Local anesthetics. *In* Barash PG, Cullen BF, Stoelting RK (eds): Clinical Anesthesia. JB Lippincott Company, Philadelphia, 1989.

Horton WG: Use of peripheral nerve stimulator. *In* Brown DL (ed): Regional Anesthesia at Virginia Mason Medical Center: A Clinical Perspective. Problems in Anesthesia Volume 1. JB Lippincott Company, Philadelphia, 1987.

McMahon D: Managing regional anesthesia equipment. *In* Brown DL (ed): Regional Anesthesia at Virginia Mason Medical Center: A Clinical Perspective. Problems in Anesthesia, Volume 1. JB Lippincott Company, Philadelphia, 1987, p 592.

Schorr MR: Needles: some points to think about. Anesth Analg 45: 509–513 (part I), 514–526 (part II), 1966.

Upper Extremity Blocks

Brown DL, Bridenbaugh LD: Physics applied to regional anesthesia results in an improved supraclavicular nerve block: The "plumb-bob" technique. Anesthesiology 69: A376, 1988.

DeJong RH: Axillary block of the brachial plexus. Anesthesiology 22: 215–225, 1961.

Finucane BT, Yilling F: Safety of supplementing axillary brachial plexus blocks. Anesthesiology 70: 401–403, 1989.

Grice SC, Morell RC, Balestrieri FJ, Stump DA, Howard G: Intravenous regional anesthesia: Evaluation and prevention of leakage under the tourniquet. Anesthesiology 65: 316–320, 1986.

Lillie PE, Glynn CJ, Fenwick DG: Site of action of intravenous regional anesthesia. Anesthesiology 61: 507–510, 1984.

Moore DC: Regional Block. 4th ed. CC Thomas, Publisher, Springfield, IL, 1965.

Partridge BL, Katz J, Benirschke K: Functional anatomy of the brachial plexus sheath: Implications for anesthesia. Anesthesiology 66: 743–747, 1987.

Peterson DO: Shoulder block anesthesia for shoulder reconstruction surgery. Anesth Analg 64: 373–375, 1985.

Sharrock NE, Bruce G: An improved technique for locating the interscalene goove. Anesthesiology 44: 431–433, 1976.

Sukhani R, Garcia CJ, Munhall RJ, Winnie AP, Rodvold KA: Lidocaine distribution following intravenous regional anesthesia with different tourniquet inflation techniques. Anesth Analg 68: 633–637, 1989.

Thompson GE, Rorie DK: Functional anatomy of the brachial plexus sheaths. Anesthesiology 59: 117–122, 1983.

Vester-Anderson T, Christiansen C, Hansen A, Sorensen M, Meisler C: Interscalene brachial plexus block: Area of analgesia, complications and blood concentrations of local anesthetics. Acta Anaesth Scand 25: 81–84, 1981.

Vester-Anderson T, Christiansen C, Sorensen M, Eriksen C: Perivascular axillary block I: Blockade following 40 ml 1% mepivacaine with adrenaline. Acta Anaesth Scand 26: 519–523, 1982.

Vester-Anderson T, Christiansen C, Sorensen M, Kaalund-Jergensen H, Saugbjerg P, Schultz-Moller K: Perivascular axillary block II: Influence of volume of local anaesthetic on neural blockade. Acta Anaesth Scand 27: 95–98, 1983.

Vester-Anderson T, Eriksen C, Christiansen C: Perivascular axillary block III: Blockade following 40 and 0.5%, 1% or 1.5% mepivacaine with adrenaline. Acta Anaesth Scand 28: 95–98, 1984.

Vester-Anderson T, Husum B, Lindeburg T, Borrits L, Gothgen I: Perivascular axillary block IV: Blockade following 40, 50 or 60 ml of mepivacaine 1% with adrenaline. Acta Anaesth Scand 28: 99–105, 1984.

Vester-Anderson T, Husum B, Lindeburg T, Borrits L, Gothgen I: Perivascular axillary block V: Blockade following 60 ml of mepivacaine 1% injected as a bolus or as 30+30ml with a 20 min interval. Acta Anaesth Scand 28: 612–616, 1984.

Vester-Anderson T, Husum B, Zaric D, Eriksen C: Perivascular axillary block VI: The effect of a supplementary dose of 20 ml mepivacaine 1% with adrenaline to patients with incomplete sensory blockade. Acta Anaesth Scand 30: 231–234, 1986.

Winnie AP: Interscalene brachial plexus block. Anesth Analg 49: 455–466, 1970.

Winnie AP: Plexus Anesthesia, Volume I: Perivascular Techniques of Brachial Plexus Block. WB Saunders Company, Philadelphia, 1983.

Lower Extremity Blocks

Beck GP: Anterior approach to sciatic nerve block. Anesthesiology 24: 222–224, 1963.

Bridenbaugh PO: The lower extremity: Somatic block. *In* Cousins M, Bridenbaugh PO (eds): Neural Blockade. 2nd ed. JB Lippincott Company, Philadelphia, 1988, pp 417–442.

Brown TCK, Dickens DRV: A new approach to lateral cutaneous nerve of thigh block. Anaesth Intensive Care 14: 126–127, 1986.

Chayen D, Nathan H, Clayen M: The psoas compartment block. Anesthesiology 45: 95–99, 1976.

Dalens B, Tanguy A, Vanneuville G: Lumbar plexus block in children. A comparison of two procedures in 50 patients. Anesth Analg 67: 750–758, 1988.

Dalens B, Tanguy A, Vanneuville G: Lumbar plexus blocks and lumbar plexus nerve blocks (letter). Anesth Analg 6: 850–857, 1989.

Dalens B, Tanguy A, Vanneuville G: Sciatic nerve block in children: Comparison of the posterior, anterior, and lateral approaches in 180 pediatric patients. Anesth Analg 70: 131–137, 1990.

Hopkins PM, Ellis FR, Halsall PJ: Evaluation of local anaesthetic blockade of the lateral femoral cutaneous nerve. Anaesthesia 46: 95–96, 1991.

Labat G: Regional Anesthesia: Its Technique and Clinical Application. WB Saunders Company, Philadelphia, 1923.

McNicol LR: Sciatic nerve block for children: anterior approach for postoperative pain relief. Anaesthesia 40: 410–414, 1985.

Moore DC: Regional Block. 4th ed. CC Thomas, Publisher, Springfield, IL, 1965.

Parkinson SK, Mueller JB, Little WL, Bailey SL: Extent of blockade with various approaches to the lumbar plexus. Anesth Analg 68: 243–248, 1989.

Rorie DK, Byer DE, Nelson DO, Sittipong R, Johnson KA: Assessment of block of the sciatic nerve in the popliteal fossa. Anesth Analg 59: 371–376, 1980.

Schurman DJ: Ankle-block anesthesia for foot surgery. Anesthesiology 44: 348–352, 1976.

Winnie AP, Ramamurthy S, Durrani Z: The inguinal paravascular technic of lumbar plexus anesthesia: The ''3-in-1'' block. Anesth Analg 52: 989–996, 1973.

Head and Neck Blocks

Barton S, Williams JD: Glossopharyngeal nerve block. Arch Otolaryngol 93: 186–188, 1971.

Bedder MD, Lindsay DL: Glossopharyngeal nerve block using ultrasound guidance: A case report of a new technique. Reg Anaesth 14: 304–307, 1989.

Feitl ME, Krupin T: Neural blockade for ophthalmologic surgery. In Cousins M, Bridenbaugh PO (eds): Neural Blockade. 2nd ed. JB Lippincott Company, Philadelphia, 1988, pp 577–592.

Eriksson E (ed): Illustrated Handbook in Local Anaesthesia. 2nd ed. WB Saunders Company, Philadelphia, 1980.

Gotta AW, Sullivan CA: Anaesthesia of the upper airway using topical anaesthetic and superior laryngeal nerve block. Br J Anaesth 53: 1055–1057, 1981.

Kroll DA, Knight PR, Mullin V: Electrocardiographic changes in patients with stellate ganglion blockade. Reg Anaesth 7: 157–159, 1982.

Macintosh RR, Ostlere M: Local Analgesia: Head and Neck. E & S Livingstone, Ltd, Edinburgh, 1955.

Moore DC: Stellate Ganglion Block. CC Thomas, Publisher, Springfield, IL, 1954.

Murphy TM: Somatic blockade of head and neck. In Cousins M, Bridenbaugh PO (eds): Neural Blockade. 2nd ed. JB Lippincott Company, Philadelphia, 1988, pp 533–558.

Winnie AP, Ramamuthy S, Durrani Z, Radonjic R: Interscalene cervical plexus block: A single injection technique. Anesth Analg 54: 370–375, 1975.

Truncal Blocks

Brown DL: Neurolytic celiac plexus block in your practice. In Brown DL (ed): Regional Anesthesia at Virginia Mason Medical Center: A Clinical Perspective. Problems in Anesthesia, Volume 1. JB Lippincott Company, Philadelphia, 1987, pp 612–621.

Bugedo GJ, Carcamo CR, Mertens RA, Dagino JA, Munoz HR: Preoperative percutaneous ilioinguinal and iliohypogastric nerve block with 0.5% bupivacaine for post-herniorrhaphy pain management in adults. Reg Anaesth 15: 130–133, 1990.

Cherry DA, Rao DM: Lumbar sympathetic and coeliac plexus blocks: An anatomical study in cadavers. Br J Anaesth 54: 1037, 1982.

Conacher ID: Resin injection of thoracic paravertebral spaces. Br J Anaesth 61: 657–661, 1988.

Covino BG: Interpleural regional anesthesia (editorial). Anesth Analg 67: 427–429, 1987.

Crossley AWA, Hosie HE: Radiographic study of intercostal nerve blockade in healthy volunteers. Br J Anaesth 59: 149–154, 1987.

Ischia S, Luzzani A, Ischia A, Faggion S: A new approach to neurolytic block of the coeliac plexus: The transaortic technique. Pain 16: 333–341, 1983.

Katz J, Renck H: Handbook of Thoraco-Abdominal Nerve Block. Grune & Stratton, Orlando, FL, 1987.

Moore DC, Bush WH, Scurlock JE: Intercostal nerve block: A roentgenographic anatomic study of technique and absorption in humans. Anesth Analg 59: 815–825, 1979.

Moore DC, Bush WH, Burnett LL: Celiac plexus block: A roentgenographic, anatomic study of technique and spread of solution in patients and corpses. Anesth Analg 60: 369–379, 1981.

Moore DC: Intercostal nerve block: Spread of India ink injected to the rib's costal groove. Br J Anaesth 53: 325–329, 1981.

Mulroy MF: Intercostal block at the mid-axillary line. Reg Anaesth 10: A39, 1985.

Rocco A, Reiestad F, Gudman J, McKay W: Intrapleural administration of local anesthetics for pain relief in patients with multiple rib fractures. Reg Anaesth 12: 10–14, 1987.

Stromskag KE, Hauge O, Steen PA: Distribution of local anesthetics injected into the interpleural space, studied by computerized tomography. Acta Anaesth Scand 34: 323–326, 1990.

Thompson GE, Brown DL: The common nerve blocks. In Nunn JF, Utting JE, Brown BR (eds): General Anaesthesia. 5th ed. Butterworth, London, 1989, pp 1049–1085.

Thompson GE, Moore DC: Celiac plexus, intercostal, and minor peripheral blockade. In Cousins M, Bridenbaugh PO (eds): Neural Blockade. 2nd ed. JB Lippincott Company, Philadelphia, 1988, pp 503–532.

Tverskoy M, Cozacov C, Ayache M, Bradely EL, Kissin I: Postoperative pain after inguinal herniorrhaphy with different types of anesthesia. Anesth Analg 70: 29–35, 1990.

Umeda S, Arai T, Hatano Y, Mori K, Hoshino K: Cadaver anatomic analysis of the best site for chemical lumbar sympathectomy. Anesth Analg 66: 643–646, 1987.

Ward EM, Rorie DK, Nauss LA, Bahn RC: The celiac ganglia in man: Normal anatomic variations. Anesth Analg 58: 461–465, 1979.

Centroneuraxis Block

Blomberg RG: A method for epiduroscopy and spinaloscopy: Presentation of preliminary results. Acta Anaesth Scand 29: 113–116, 1985.

Blomberg RG: The dorsomedian connective tissue band in the lumbar epidural space of humans: An anatomic study using epiduroscopy in autopsy cases. Anesth Analg 65: 747–752, 1986.

Blomberg RG: The lumbar subdural extraarachnoid space in of humans: An anatomical study using spinaloscopy in autopsy cases. Anesth Analg 66: 177–180, 1987.

Blomberg RG, Olsson SS: The lumbar epidural space in patients examined with epiduroscopy. Anesth Analg 68: 157–160, 1989.

Bridenbaugh PO, Greene NM: Spinal (subarachnoid) neural blockade. In Cousins M, Bridenbaugh PO (eds): Neural Blockade. 2nd ed. JB Lippincott Company, Philadelphia, 1988, pp 213–251.

Bromage PR: Epidural Anesthesia. WB Saunders Company, Philadelphia, 1978.

Brown DL, Wedel DJ: Spinal, epidural and caudal anesthesia. In Miller RD (ed): Anesthesia. 3rd ed. Churchill Livingstone, New York, 1990, pp 1377–1405.

Brown EM, Elman DS: Postoperative backache. Anesth Analg 40: 683–685,1961.

Butler BD, Warters RD, Elk JR, Davies I, Abouleish E: Loss of resistance technique for locating the epidural space: Evaluation of glass and plastic syringes. Can J Anaesth 37: 438–439, 1990.

Caldwell C, Nielsen C, Baltz T, Taylor P, Helton B, Butler P: Comparison of high-dose epinephrine and phenylephrine in spinal anesthesia with tetracaine. Anesthesiology 62: 804–807, 1985.

Concepcion M, Maddi R, Francis D, Rocco AG, Murray E, Covino BG: Vasoconstrictors in spinal anesthesia with tetracaine: A comparison of epinephrine and phenylephrine. Anesth Analg 63: 134–138, 1984.

Cousins MJ, Bromage PR: Epidural neural blockade. In Cousins M, Bridenbaugh PO (eds): Neural Blockade. 2nd ed. JB Lippincott Company, Philadelphia, 1988, pp 253–360.

Covino BG, Scott DB: Handbook of Epidural Anaesthesia and Analgesia. Grune & Stratton, Orlando, FL, 1985.

DiGiovanni AJ, Dunbar BS: Epidural injections of autologous blood for post-lumbar puncture headache. Anesth Analg 49: 268–271, 1970.

Gallart L, Blanco D, Samso E, Vidal F: Clinical and radiologic evidence of the epidural plica mediana dorsalis. Anesth Analg 71: 698–701, 1990.

Gormley JB: Treatment of postspinal headache. Anesthesiology 21: 565–566, 1960.

Greene NM: Physiology of Spinal Anesthesia. 3rd ed. Williams & Wilkins, Baltimore, 1981.

Greene NM: Distribution of local anesthetic solutions within the subarachnoid space. Anesth Analg 64: 715–730, 1985.

Greene NM: Uptake and elimination of local anesthetics during spinal anesthesia. Anesth Analg 62: 1013–1024, 1983.

Hardy PAJ: Can epidural catheters penetrate dura matter? An anatomical study. Anaesthesia 41: 1146–1147, 1986.

Harrison GR, Clowes NWB: The depth of the lumbar epidural space from the skin. Anaesthesia 40: 685–687, 1985.

Kane RE: Neurologic deficits following epidural or spinal anesthesia. Anesth Analg 60: 150–161, 1981.

Kozody R, Palahniuk RJ, Wade JG, Cumming MO: The effect of subarachnoid epinephrine and phenylephrine on spinal cord blood flow. Can Anaesth Soc J 31: 503–508, 1984.

Leicht CH, Carlson SA: Prolongation of lidocaine spinal anesthesia with epinephrine and phenylephrine. Anesth Analg 65: 365–369, 1986.

Lund PC: Reflections upon the historical aspects of spinal anesthesia. Reg Anaesth 8: 89–98, 1983.

Marinacci AA: Neurologic aspects of complications of spinal anesthesia. LA Neurol Soc Bull 25: 170–192, 1960.

Meiklejohn BH: Distance from skin to the lumbar epidural space in obstetric population. Reg Anaesth 15: 134–136, 1990.

Moore DC: Regional Block. 4th ed. CC Thomas, Publisher, Springfield, IL, 1965.

Moore DC, Bridenbaugh LD: Spinal (subarachnoid) block: A review of 11,574 cases. JAMA 195: 907–912, 1966.

Moore DC, Bridenbaugh LD, Bagdi PA, Bridenbaugh PO, Stander H: The present status of spinal (subarachnoid) and epidural (peridural) block. Anesth Analg 47: 40–49, 1968.

Moore DC: Spinal anesthesia: Bupivacaine compared with tetracaine. Anesth Analg 59: 743–750, 1980.

Moore DC, Chadwick HS, Ready LB: Epinephrine prolongs lidocaine spinal: Pain in the operative site: the most accurate method of determining local anesthetic duration. Anesthesiology 67: 416–418, 1987.

Reynolds AF, Roberts PA, Pollay M, Stratemeier PH: Quantitative anatomy of the thoracolumbar epidural space. Neurosurgery 17: 905–907, 1985.

Rigler ML, Drasner K, Krejcie TC, Yelich SJ, Scholnick FT, DeFontes J, Bohner D: Cauda equina syndrome after continuous spinal anesthesia. Anesth Analg 72: 275–281, 1991.

Savolaine ER, Pandya JB, Greenblatt SH, Conover SR: Anatomy of the human lumbar epidural space: New insights using CT-epidurography. Anesthesiology 68: 217–220, 1988.

Smith TC: The lumbar spine and subarachnoid block. Anesthesiology 29: 60–64, 1968.

Tarkkila PJ: Incidence and causes of failed spinal anesthetics in a university hospital: A prospective study. Reg Anaesth 16: 48–51, 1991.

Taylor JA: Lumbosacral subarachnoid tap. J Urol 43: 561–564, 1940.

Trotter M: Variations of the sacral canal: Their significance in the administration of caudal anesthesia. Anesth Analg 26: 192–202, 1947.

Tuominen M: Bupivacaine spinal anaesthesia. Acta Anaesth Scand 35: 1–10, 1991.

Vandam LD, Dripps RD: A long-term follow-up of patients who received 10,098 spinal anesthetics. II: Incidence and analyses of minor sensory neurologic defects. Surgery 38: 463–469, 1955.

Willis RJ: Caudal epidural block. *In* Cousins M, Bridenbaugh PO (eds): Neural Blockade. 2nd ed. JB Lippincott Company, Philadelphia, 1988, pp 361–383.

Zarzur E: Anatomic studies of the human lumbar ligamentum flavum. Anesth Analg 63: 499–502, 1984.

Index

Note: Page numbers in *italics* refer to illustrations.